PRIVATISATION AND SOCIAL POLICY

Longman Social Policy in Britain series

Series editor: Jo Campling

Books already published in the series:

Health Policy and the NHS: Towards 2000 *Second edition*
J.M. Allsop

Housing Problems and Housing Policy
Brian Lund

Personal Social Services: Clients, Consumers or Citizens?
Robert Adams

The Foundations of the Welfare State
Pat Thane

Older People in Modern Society
Anthea Tinker

Responding to Poverty: The Politics of Cash and Care
Saul Becker

Equal Opportunities and Social Policy: Issues of Gender, Race and Disability
B. Bagilhole

Disabled People and Social Policy: From Exclusion to Inclusion
M.J. Oliver

Privatisation and Social Policy
Mark Drakeford

PRIVATISATION AND SOCIAL POLICY

MARK DRAKEFORD

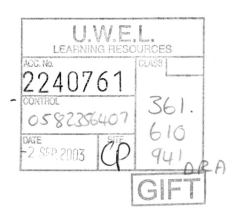
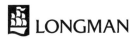 LONGMAN

An imprint of **PEARSON EDUCATION**

Harlow, England · London · New York · Reading, Massachusetts · San Francisco · Toronto · Don Mills, Ontario · Sydney
Tokyo · Singapore · Hong Kong · Seoul · Taipei · Cape Town · Madrid · Mexico City · Amsterdam · Munich · Paris · Milan

Pearson Education Limited
Edinburgh Gate
Harlow
Essex CM20 2JE
England
and Associated Companies throughout the world

Visit us on the World Wide Web at:
www.pearsoned-ema.com

First published 2000

ISBN 0–582–35640–7 PPR

British Library Cataloguing-in-Publication Data

A catalogue record for this book is
available from the British Library

Set by 35 in Baskerville

Printed in Malaysia,LSP

CONTENTS

Contents

PREFACE

I am very pleased to provide the preface for Mark Drakeford's *Privatisation and Social Policy*. He has produced a work that is both stimulating and challenging while being accessible to the intelligent lay reader. As other authors know, this is no mean feat. The book itself draws on and develops themes that have represented a significant part of the author's work over the last decade. Indeed, I think that it is true to say that Drakeford's work over the last ten years embodies some of the most interesting social policy literature both on how the socially excluded experience social exclusion and how social policies contribute to their exclusion. This volume picks up these and other themes and concentrates on the de-nationalisation or privatisation of the welfare state. This process is carefully analysed in relation to each of the welfare state services in the latter part of the book but is prefaced by a theoretical and analytical discussion of where privatisation comes from, what it means and what its effects are and are likely to be. Together, the discussion and the analysis provide salutary lessons for policy-makers and practitioners alike and contribute to make a textbook of the highest quality. But this is not just a textbook. Through the use of his own and other writers' research, Drakeford takes the debate forward. He traces the origins of the privatisation of social policy to the social policies, and more importantly, the economic and political principles of neo-liberal Conservatism. But he also considers how such policies form part of a sort of Blairite 'Third Way'.

The author's project is addressed with both a dispassionate eye and a passionate (or compassionate) heart. And the book is the better for the marriage of the two. This is a book on the welfare state, written by someone who can rightly be regarded an academic expert. It is also a book about social policy written by an author who ardently believes in the capacity of social policy to ameliorate social ills and knows its capacity, also, to contribute to their exacerbation. It is to be recommended to all who wish to understand the social policy of the late Twentieth Century.

Michael Sullivan
Swansea
June 1999

LIST OF ABBREVIATIONS

APS	Assisted Places Scheme
ASBO	Anti-Social Behaviour Order
AST	Advanced Skills Teacher
BPU	Budget Payment Unit
CBI	Confederation of British Industries
CCT	Compulsory Competitive Tendering
CSR	Comprehensive Spending Review
CTC	City Technology College
DoE	Department of the Environment
DES	Department of Education and Science
DETR	Department of the Environment, Transport and the Regions
DfE/WO	Department for Education (Welsh Office)
DFEE	Department of Education and Employment
DoH	Department of Health
DHA	District Health Authority
DHSS	Department of Health and Social Security
DSS	Department of Social Security
EAZ	Education Action Zone
ERCF	Estates Renewal Challenge Fund
GM	Grant Maintained
GP	General Practitioner
GPCG	General Practitioner Commissioning Group
GPFH	General Practioner Fundholder
HAT	Housing Action Trust
HSSSSAA	Health and Social Services and Social Security Adjudications Act
JRF	Joseph Rowntree Foundation
JSA	Job Seekers Allowance
LEA	Local Education Authority
LSVT	Large Scale Voluntary Transfer
MIRAS	Mortgage Interest Tax Relief
NCB	National Children's Bureau
NHS	National Health Service
OFSTED	The Office for Standards in Education
OFT	Office of Fair Trading

PCG	Primary Care Group
PFI	Private Finance Initiative
PSBR	Public Sector Borrowing Requirement
REC	Regional Electricity Company
RTB	Right to Buy
SCAA	Schools Curriculum Assessment Authority
SERPS	State Earnings Related Pension Scheme
SEU	Social Exclusion Unit
SSD	Social Services Department
STG	Special Transitional Grant

ACKNOWLEDGEMENTS

This book is the product of an idea which has been a personal preoccupation ever since becoming involved in the investigation of the social consequences of the privatised utilities in Wales. I'm especially grateful, therefore, to those colleagues in the anti-poverty movement here who have provided so much of the impetus to bring these findings and ideas to a wider audience. While working at Swansea – where this work began – I was particularly encouraged by Mike Sullivan to think more widely about the impact of privatisation upon social welfare services. He has remained willing, ever since, to be a sounding-board for work-in-progress and I want to record my continuing appreciation of that help and the Preface which he has now contributed to this volume.

The main debt which I owe, in bringing the project to publication lies unambiguously with Jo Campling from whose advice and thoughtfulness. I have been the grateful beneficiary. This book would not have happened without it – or, indeed, the consistent helpfulness of Verina Pettigrew and other staff at Longman.

Families bear the worst brunt of the pressures which preparing manuscripts entails. I've been more than lucky to have the active help of my father, John, and my wife, Clare, in bringing this book to publication.

Errors of fact, infelicities of expression, peculiarities of interpretation, perversities of conclusion – all these, of course, remain entirely my own responsibility.

Mark Drakeford
Cardiff
June 1999

PART ONE

Chapter 1

INTRODUCTION

This is a book concerned with one of the great debates of contemporary social policy, and one which is older than the discipline itself. Defining the boundary between public and private responsibility was a part of Plato's debates about the nature of state and citizenship. It framed the Elizabethan resolution of parish provision for the poor and determined the founding instrument of the modern welfare state, the Poor Law Amendment Act of 1834. Even in periods when the balance between those responsibilities assumed by the state and those undertaken by individuals has appeared stable and decided, an undercurrent of dissent, disagreement and ambition for alternative arrangements lies closer to the surface than casual enquiry might suggest.

For almost two centuries, however, these changing balances have taken place within an overall pattern in which the collective organisations of societies and states have taken an increasing responsibility for the welfare of individuals. The achievement of a 'welfare state' – even where marked by reluctance rather than enthusiasm, and by self-interest rather than altruism – provides a deep current over which particular ebbs and flows of public and private provision have taken place. For a text concerned with *privatisation* this deep pattern is particularly important. It gives rise to the immediate question of whether the ambition of 'rolling back the state', which has characterised British social policy during the last quarter of the twentieth century, is another temporary disturbance upon the face of the ocean, or whether it amounts, really, to a sea-change in welfare thinking and organisation.

Within our own time, certainty regarding these basic issues of social policy has been largely overtaken, both by debate about the particular issue of public and private provision and by the general post-modernist emphasis upon uncertainty and risk. Among the political parties it has become common ground that change in the provision of welfare, its costs, the services it provides, the rights and obligations which it confers upon individual citizens and so on is inevitable. Here are two views, one expressed by the deputy leader of his Party, the other by the leader of his – 'There is no escaping the need for structural reforms of the social security system' and 'We have reached the limits of the public's willingness simply to fund an unreformed welfare state through ever higher taxes and spending.' The first expresses the view of Peter Lilley, the second that of Tony Blair. The characterisation of welfare as a problem unites both views.

The solution to that problem, of course, is a matter of contention and contradiction. Part of the purpose of this book will be to place present-day debates in the context of longer-term concerns, attempting to connect these dilemmas to the discussions from which they have sprung.

It will also be a purpose, however, to suggest a particular understanding of those currents which appear to be running most strongly in contemporary welfare and to consider their impact upon those by whom social welfare services are required. Even if disputing the dividing line between private and public provision turns out, on examination, to be a continuous thread in this area of policy, that continuity should not obscure the very real differences which boundary changes create for individuals and whole classes of individuals. Nor should the time-honoured nature of these debates prevent us from remaining alert to the possibility that even continuous spectrums could have paradigm shifts within them, in which the balance might shift – even temporarily – between significantly different elements.

For students of social policy, these questions lie at the core of their discipline. The ambition of this text is to provide some of the information and argument which allows debate around that core to be conducted. While I make no claim to neutrality in drawing conclusions in this ideologically contested terrain, my aim has been to remain as explicit as possible about my own interpretation, thus allowing readers to reach quite different conclusions, where these appear to them to be more convincing.

1.1 Structure of the book

The structure of the text may be summarised as follows. Part One places contemporary controversies concerning privatisation and marketisation in the longer-term context of such debates within social welfare. Chapter 2 aims to set out the case for increasing the scope of private provision and market organisation in terms which would be recognisable to those who espouse such views. Chapter 3 discusses the practical application of privatisation and marketisation policies in an area where promoters of such polices have made greatest claims – the privatised utilities. This chapter explores the social policy consequences of initiatives which were advanced primarily on industrial and economic grounds. A set of issues emerge as relevant to social policy services more widely and these are considered in the subject-by-subject chapters which make up Part Two of the book. This section deals with the period of Conservative government between 1979 and 1997, when such policies occupied an unambiguous place on the agenda of administration. Part Three turns to the emerging record of the New Labour government, elected in May 1997. The application of private and public solutions to social policy problems by the Blair administration will be recorded and assessed. The final part – Part Four – provides a series of key documents, setting out the ideological framework within which privatisation and marketisation policies are derived and disputed and setting out the claims made for and against such policies in their application to social welfare services.

In as complex an area as privatisation and marketisation of social welfare services, it will not be possible to provide equal attention to all the possible techniques, approaches and claims made for them in the case of each policy area. Instead, the plan adopted in this book has been to provide a particular emphasis within each service chapter, illustrating and exploring the application of particular techniques and evaluating the outcomes. Of course, this does not preclude each chapter considering other relevant applications; nor does it prevent an aspect which has received concentrated consideration in one area from appearing again in another. It does provide a means, however, by which the most important elements in the application of privatisation in social welfare can receive the attention required.

It is in the nature of the social policy issues considered in this book that individual chapters must deal with the application of macro-level policies created by governments at the meso-level of particular services. The impact of privatisation and marketisation, however, is not simply felt at a service level. Users of particular forms of social policy provision are directly affected by the changes outlined. As Papadakis and Taylor-Gooby (1987: 32) put it, 'reduction in state involvement in any service to meet need involves the expansion of the private sector, because people are compelled to meet their needs privately, if they can'. Each chapter, therefore, also includes an investigation of change at an individual level, providing most attention to the impact of privatisation upon those most in need of services. Moran (1998: 30) suggests that, 'market ideology simultaneously holds out prospects of empowerment and of subordination'. The case made by privatisers and marketeers concentrates heavily upon the former, and this book will provide a series of examples where empowerment has taken place – patients able to buy access to medical care; parents able to obtain a school place of choice; and so on. However, the sharpest test of a policy has to be among the hardest cases and it will be in this area, which Moran characterises as subordination, that each chapter will deal at its conclusion.

This introductory chapter aims to trace some of the boundary shifts which have taken place in the five core social policy areas with which this text is primarily concerned. Individual chapters will later consider the impact of privatisation and marketisation upon these services from 1979 onwards. Here I aim to present the balance between private and public provision in housing, education, social security, social services and health at the end of the 1970s, providing the context within which later changes can be understood. The end of this chapter will return to the more general question of what is meant by the term 'privatisation' in this book, leading into an account of its modern policy development and its application.

Housing

Chapter 4, dealing with housing policy, places particular emphasis upon the privatisation of property in social welfare, tracing the direct transfer of material goods and assets – primarily council housing – from the public to the private spheres. While state acceptance of responsibility for housing has never, as in the case of education or health, been undertaken on a universal basis, the flow of policy during the first eighty years of this century was almost always in that direction. Immediately after the First World War the pressure to provide homes for returning heroes resulted in government subsidy to private house builders in order to encourage production. Government thus used its financial power to buy services – in this case house building – provided by others. In this way, the system represented an early example of the provider/purchaser division which was to be a central technique of the 1980s free marketeers. Nor, as Hendry (1998: 15) notes, were these the first attempts at such a policy. Unsuccessful attempts to provide local authorities with financial assistance to build working-class homes had been introduced in Parliament in 1912, 1913 and again in 1914. While the Addison Act of 1919 established the effectiveness of government subsidy in stimulating private production of housing, it also allowed for the direct provision of housing by local government where the need for this could be demonstrated. While only 75,900 local authority houses were built under the Addison arrangements, as opposed to 362,000 by the private sector (Hendry 1998: 18), the principle of direct state provision had been established. The Wheatley Act of the 1924 Labour government led to the construction of half a million local authority dwellings in less than a decade. Thereafter, while the scale of subsidy and construction varied at different periods, the fact of state intervention and provision had been achieved, albeit within a market in which most people would remain housed within the private sectors of renting and house purchase.

For the greater part of the twentieth century, involvement of the state in housing policy rested essentially upon twin foundations. On the one hand, housing was, as Linneman and Megbolugbe (1994: 641) suggest, 'always re-garded as a "merit" good. The provision of a decent home for every family was generally considered part of the basic responsibility of government.' The case for assuming such a responsibility drew on the intrinsic importance of decent accommodation – the fact that, as Balchin and Rhoden (1998: xvii) put it, 'apart from nourishment, shelter is humankind's most essential material need'. Less altruistically, state interest also rested upon the 'externalities' of housing – that is to say, the way in which the consequences of failure to provide decent housing might impact upon those indirectly, as well as directly, affected through, for example, the spread of disease. Direct involvement of government in achiev-ing such an end, however, was relatively constrained. Smith *et al.* (1996: 288) set this in the context of other social policy areas: 'Unlike education or health service provision there has never been a commitment on the part of any gov-ernment, of whatever political persuasion, to support a near universal housing service designed to meet the needs of all households.' Rather, state intervention was confined to a redistribution of housing resources towards poorer citizens, bringing decent and affordable accommodation within the reach of those who would otherwise be unable to obtain access to it. Regulation of the private rented market and direct provision of council housing have been the primary means through which this outcome has been sought. While local authority housing, as a proportion of the total housing stock, reached its peak in 1978 (Hills 1991), Forrest (1993: 40) argues that, in most localities, 'it was the private sector which was the dominant provider either through mortgaged owner-occupation or private renting'. The importance of the private sector, moreover, was common currency between the political parties by the end of the 1970s. Williams (1992: 161), for example, notes that the Housing Review undertaken by the Labour government between 1975 and 1977,

> 'asserted the importance of home ownership and proposed no changes to MIRAS . . . In 1978 the Labour government introduced its new Housing Bill. This included . . . measures to extend home ownership and improve the allocation of council housing . . . much of this was taken up by the Conservatives when they returned to power in 1979 and introduced their own Housing Bill.'

It is in response to such evidence that Malpass (1998: 186) concludes that, 'the changes imposed in the 1980s and those planned in the 1990s are rooted in trends that were well established before 1979'.

At the same time, the impetus for privatisation and marketisation from 1979 onwards was, in many ways, driven by financial as well as ideological considerations. The welfare state of the post-war period was, in many ways, a local state. Of the great services considered in this book, three – education, housing, social services – remained the province of local councils, while two – the health service and social security – were organised on a national basis. The growth in local government spending on welfare services fuelled this concern. Butcher (1995: 92–3) shows that local authority expenditure, as a proportion of total public spending, had risen from about one-quarter at the end of the 1940s to nearly one-third by 1976.

Within that picture, spending on education, housing and the personal social services had risen from 24 per cent of local government spending in 1945 to nearly 62 per cent in 1976. The arrival of the oil crisis and the consequent economic recession of the mid-1970s brought that era of expansion to an end. The Conservative Party analysis of the economic crisis of the mid and late 1970s was one which identified public spending as a cause of national difficulty, rather than a solution to problems of the state. It thus prepared the ground for privatisation as a key part of the general attack on the scope of state activity. It was against this general background, therefore, that the 1979 Conservative Government entered office with a more developed approach in relation to housing than in almost all other social policy areas. It intended to privatise property in the hands of the state, through the sale of local authority houses to council tenants. In doing so, however, it was operating within a field in which pluralism and the co-existence of public and private had long been characteristic.

Social security

Chapter 5, devoted to social security, will look in detail at the phenomenon known as 'privatising from within' (Young 1986: 243), in which private sector techniques – or 'new public management' doctrines – are applied to public sector services. Market-testing and the creation of government agencies will form the focus of re-delineating the boundary between public and private provision. The relief or prevention of poverty through income maintenance policies is one of the most fundamental parts of the contract between the citizen and the state. Chapter 5 considers the changing balance of rights and responsibilities within that relationship inherent in the application of privatisation and marketisation to social security policy.

The particular concerns of Chapter 5 thus have to be understood in the wider context of the development of British social security policy. The distinction between responsibilities to be accepted by the state, and those to be undertaken by the individual, has been more sharply felt in relation to the provision of income than in any other social policy area considered in this text. A minimal system, consistent with the prevention of social unrest, has been a recurring theme here, together with a consistent preoccupation to make the lives of those dependent upon a state-provided income no more comfortable than those of the least well off in employment. This latter principle of 'less-eligibility' found its most powerful expression in the Poor Law Amendment Act of 1834 which set the framework for more than a century of social security provision. At least partly as a result of the hardship caused by that Act, the nineteenth century witnessed the development of a large-scale 'self-help' sector, made up of trades unions, friendly societies, building societies and others through which, as Hill (1990: 17) suggests, individual self-help could be supported and sustained by collective effort.

In so far as the state intruded upon private provision during the nineteenth century, this effort consisted of attempts to regulate and formalise, rather than supplant, the voluntary and commercial sectors. Even this limited activity, however, proved controversial. Doran (1994) has traced the opposition of the late eighteenth-century 'Box Clubs' to requirements that their system of voluntary contributions and benefits to members might be overseen by professional actuaries. The Clubs were alert to suggestions, made in Parliament at the end of the Napoleonic Wars, that the burden of poor relief upon parishes might be reduced by making membership of friendly societies compulsory. Doran (1994: 139) quotes a contribution recorded in *Hansard* of 1819, that:

> 'Many persons thought this mode of providing the wants of the poor so desirable, that its operation ought not to be left to the voluntary acts of individuals, but that the poor should be compelled to resort to it.' (*Hansard*, vol. 39: 1819: 1160–1)

Despite these objections, however, the trend towards greater formality within self-help organisations continued, providing the respectable working class with a form of insurance against both the dangers of unemployment and ill-health and against the necessity of relying upon the deterrent assistance afforded by the state. Increased casualisation of employment, however, and a growing electorate combined to provide the first major shift in favour of a state-provided social security system. The Old Age Pensions Act of 1908 and the ill-health and unemployment benefits of the 1911 National Insurance Act established the framework of the system which remained in place throughout the inter-war period. By the time of the 1942 Beveridge Report, the social security system remained a complex mixture of public and private provision. Within the state system, an insurance-based scheme provided for most people on low and middle incomes in relation to sickness, unemployment and old age. This system was accompanied by a much despised means-tested scheme for those beyond the scope of insurance and backed up by the threat of the workhouse for those unwilling or unable to bring themselves within the scope of outdoor relief. For those in better paid employment, or wishing to secure themselves against additional hazards, the voluntary and commercial insurance markets continued to provide a private route to social security. To quote just one example, it has been estimated that, by 1938, there were more than 100 million insurance policies intended to provide help with funeral payments current in Britain (Calvert 1978: 248). These policies were held with friendly societies and commercial insurance companies. They provided minimal coverage, but sufficient to 'avoid a pauper's funeral' (Fraser 1984: 165). In fact, as Brown (1995: 16) suggests, prior to national insurance, these policies continued to represent 'the buoyant part of the market' as far as the companies were concerned. State 'interference' in provision had long been resisted by them, as part of the continuing controversy concerning the boundary between individual and collective responsibility.

The communal sacrifices of wartime conditions, however, provided a decisive twist to the debate between public and private provision. The power of the state to wage war could be harnessed in peacetime to wage war upon Beveridge's Five Giants: Want, Disease, Ignorance, Squalor and Idleness. It is not part of the purpose of this text to provide a detailed account of the achievements and limitations of the Beveridge settlement. In terms of the shifting boundary between private and public responsibility, however, the report, and the legislative programme which followed, placed its emphasis firmly upon the role of the state to organise and provide a system of National Insurance, in which all citizens would be protected from want, as of right, from the cradle to the grave *[document 1]* this, and all other documents, can be found in Chapter 11. The system, as characterised by Webb *et al.* (1976: 7) was to be 'comprehensive and universal, professional and impartial'. To pursue the example provided above in relation to funeral expenses, Beveridge suggested replacing the complicated, overlapping and inadequate benefits available through private insurance with a universal Death Grant. It was to be set at £20 for each adult, a sum which was 'reasonable to meet the necessary expenses of a decent funeral' (Beveridge 1942: 159).

If £20 would be insufficient, wrote Beveridge (1942: 159), 'there would be no difficulty in providing a larger grant'. The power of the state to provide for individual need was unchangeable.

Yet, within a very short period the first signs of challenge were beginning to become apparent. Within the complex history of income maintenance in Britain in the period from 1945 to 1979 a small number of trends need to be identified if the position to which the privatising policies of the 1980s and 1990s were applied is to be properly understood. Firstly, the system of universal contributions and benefits, as envisaged by Beveridge, did not succeed in replacing the means-tested element within social security, as he had envisaged. Universal benefits were never set at a sufficiently high level to provide for even basic needs and, as a result, and despite successive attempts in 1955, 1966 and 1974–76 to re-establish the universal basis of the scheme, means-testing grew inexorably. By the time of the first Thatcher administration, the outgoing Labour government had explicitly accepted the role which means-testing would play in the future development of social security. The 1978 nil-cost Orme Review of supplementary benefits was designed to fit that part of the system for 'its new mass role'. At the same time, at an administrative level, increasingly stringent tests of eligibility policed access to such benefits more and more tightly. The Orme Report was available for incoming Conservative Ministers and helped shape their early social security reforms, as Chapter 5 demonstrates.

At the same time, the preoccupation with the public welfare system of income maintenance was challenged by Titmuss's famous 1955 analysis of the social division of welfare, in which he drew attention to the enduring importance of fiscal and occupational contributions to social security (in Titmuss 1958). The inadequacy of national insurance-based pensions, for example, meant that, from the outset, the state system was unable to provide a universal pension in old age which would be sufficient to support a reasonable lifestyle. In the years between 1945 and 1979, a dual system developed in which the relatively well-off made private provision while the poorest were obliged to draw upon means-tested benefits, as well as the basic pension, in order to meet everyday needs. Fawcett (1995: 153) traces the change in private occupational pension coverage which grew from 13 per cent in 1936 to 33 per cent in 1955 and had come to cover approximately half the workforce by 1979. This growth was positively promoted by Conservative administrations throughout this whole period, using the tax system – Titmuss's fiscal welfare – to encourage private provision in social security.

By 1979, therefore, the universal, rights-based, adequate system of state-provided social security was already significantly in retreat. The shift from insurance-based to means-tested benefits carried within it a parallel shift from state to individual responsibility. More generally, the private provision of occupational welfare – private pensions, private health care, company cars, subsidised canteens and so on – had begun to create a more attractive alternative set of social security rights for those in employment. At the start of the 1980s the shifting balance between public and private provision was as open to amendment in this policy area as in any other.

Education

Chapter 6, dealing with education policy, focuses upon the issues of competition and choice in social welfare, exploring these questions in relation to the creation of a market between schools in the public sector. The privatising and marketising policies of the last decades of this century have to be viewed against the increasing assumption of public responsibility for education which had been in progress for more than 150 years. The first grant made by the state in education took place in 1833 when £20,000 was provided to two national voluntary bodies, the National Society of the Church of England and the Nonconformist British and Foreign Bible Society. Once again, the state was the purchaser of services provided by others. This preference for private provision remained characteristic until the latter part of the century, although government funding of private institutions – on a per capita basis, combined with payment-by-results and an attendance element which pre-figured the formula-funding of school budgets at the end of the twentieth century – grew from 1833 onwards.

The Education Act of 1870 introduced the first direct state provision of education, with 'Board schools' set up in areas where voluntary and private sector provision had failed to meet demand for elementary education. Present-day free-market liberals have suggested that investigation of the 'impressive collection of agencies outside the formal state education system, paid by parents, grandparents, employers, charities and other private sources' makes it 'clear' that educational provision would have 'continued and strengthened' had the state not intervened in the 1870 Act (West 1996: 18). When local education authorities were established under the Education Act of 1902, these were charged with aiding or directly supplying education beyond the elementary stages. Hendry (1998: 11) shows that, for the first time, the 1902 Act firmly established a 'bias towards public provision' of education, a bias which was further extended and consolidated during the inter-war period. Such was the extent of public responsibility in this field that the 1944 Education Act, while highly significant in an organisational sense, required little addition to the principle of a public responsibility for the funding and provision of a universal education service. In Hendry's analysis (1998: 14), education exemplifies a general model in the move from private to public in social policy provision over this period. The pattern begins with the introduction of public subsidy into essentially private systems. The level of this subsidy increases in order to fill gaps in private provision. Thereafter, Hendry suggests, 'once established the public sector with its great taxing powers gradually expands at the expense of private and not-for-profit sectors'. With the foundation of the welfare state, the service was effectively nationalised, provided on a universal and free-at-the-point-of-use basis. Public provision had become dominant, with private education relegated to a marginal and minority interest.

Despite the durability of this basic pattern of state responsibility, the education system which the incoming Thatcher government inherited in 1979 was one in which a number of the fundamental assumptions of the wartime Butler

Education Act of 1944 had already been strongly called into question. From within the Labour government of 1974, the Prime Minister, James Callaghan, had launched a 'Great Debate' in education, casting doubt upon the extent to which young people were equipped by it to meet the needs of industry and employment. His Ruskin speech also challenged the validity of 'child-centred' educational methods as set out in the 1943 White Paper which preceded the Butler Act. There it had been set out plainly that, 'The keynote of the new system will be that the child is the centre of education and that, so far as it is humanly possible, all children should receive the type of education to which they are best adapted.' Personal development, rather than vocational preparation, lay at the heart of the Act, and the individual child was placed at the centre of its operation. Taylor-Gooby (1993: 104) summarises the fundamental departures from those principles which the Ruskin speech embodied. It set up, he argues, 'responsiveness to the wishes of consumers and to the presumed needs of industry' as the 'touchstone by which schooling is to be judged . . . Professional judgements are swept aside: the views of those outside the educational experts' consensus – politicians, employers, parents and voters – become paramount.'

While Prime Minister Callaghan hoped to bring about a change in the delivery of education at classroom level, he remained – as he wrote 15 years later (Callaghan 1992: 16), quoting R.H. Tawney, 'what a good parent would wish for their children, so the State must wish for all its children' – a firm believer in the role of the government in pursuing such outcomes. By 1979, however, this and other basic principles of the 1944 Act were also under significant scrutiny, emanating mainly from the embryonic 'New Right' of liberal marketeers within the Conservative Party. This group, primarily in a series of publications which came to be known as the Black Papers, pointed to the enduring failure of the 1944 system to advance the interests of the most disadvantaged pupils within the education system. An Act which, as Ranson (1990: 5) suggests, had organised and legitimised itself upon claims to justice and fairness, turned out, in the argument of the Black Paper authors, to have delivered neither. In particular, the comprehensive education system, with its emphasis upon social planning and communal rather than individual preference, was attacked for the damage which it was said to have caused to educational standards and for the attack which it represented upon individual freedom. The solutions to be applied were characteristic of the New Right thinkers. The general enthusiasms of the approach was summed up by Sir Keith Joseph, soon to be Minister of Education in the cabinet of his protégé, Mrs Thatcher, in this way:

'The blind, unplanned, uncoordinated wisdom of the market is overwhelmingly superior to the well-researched, rational, systematic, well-meaning, co-operative, science-based, forward-looking, statistically respectable plans of governments, bureaucracies and international organisations.' (Joseph and Sumption 1979: 57)

Within the field of education, specifically, the advantages to be derived were later summed up by one of the co-authors of several of the Black Papers, Caroline (Lady) Cox (1988), when suggesting that, 'choice and accountability are key concepts of Conservative philosophy which underpin current educational policy. They can be the means of giving good schools the opportunity to become better; but more importantly, they can give greater power and influence to those parents and pupils who are the most vulnerable and for whom the present system is failing. Power to the people. Fairer and more democratic policies. These are our concerns.'

Thus, while education appears to be a field in which the move towards public funding of a public service had gained a firm ascendancy, the dispute between public and private remained more lively and open to question than might be apparent at first inspection. The privatisers and free-marketeers of the 1980s and 1990s were able to draw upon a tradition of dissent and alternative thinking which, as Chapter 6 illustrates, were capable of being translated into policy actions.

Social services

In considering the field of social services, Chapter 7 will devote attention to the contracting out of services which were previously provided directly by public authorities and the development of distinctive purchaser and provider roles and relationships. It will also deal closely with the question of user charges, considering the transference of responsibilities for paying for services from the public to the private sphere.

In common with all the great social welfare areas considered in this text, the personal social services had, since their inception, been subject to change in the balance between public and private responsibility in their development, funding and delivery. State intervention in the form of directly financed and provided social services, however, developed more slowly here than in any of the other policy areas. The nineteenth-century attitude towards those experiencing social problems such as poor housing, or personal difficulties such as mental illness, was that these were caused by personal inadequacy. As a result, one of the great tributary streams of modern social work – the Charity Organisation Society – was constantly preoccupied with the dangers of creating welfare dependency among its recipients. Octavia Hill, the founding genius of the Society, regarded the public provision of any 'necessary of life' to the poor as a 'disastrous policy' (Whelan 1998: 35). Towards the end of her life, as a member of the 1905 Royal Commission on the Poor Law, she submitted a memorandum of dissent to the Commission's findings in which she objected to its recommendation of free medical treatment for the poor and the idea that government might have a role in providing employment during times of economic recession. The notion of social services as the preserve of voluntary effort, selectively directed towards those who might benefit from improvement of their moral, rather than physical, circumstances remained powerful throughout the inter-war period.

The creation of modern social services departments can be traced to the 1948 Beveridge Report titled, significantly, *Voluntary Action*. Adams (1996: 31) describes this as 'the weakest of the three Beveridge Reports, but one which, nevertheless, established the idea of state responsibility for personal social services, through local authority health and welfare departments. The National Assistance Act of 1948 placed an obligation upon local councils to set up children's committees and to employ professional children's officers. The 'accepted way of thinking' about the delivery of post-1945 services – that they 'should be both financed and provided by an agency of the state' (Glennerster 1992: 31) – thus manifested itself in the social services arena. While the state had progressively come to provide the funding to support voluntary effort in the social services, the post-war priority attached to issues of equity and accountability meant that the roles of funder and provider were merged into one. Social services departments, for example, would finance the residential care of older people and provide that care directly in council-run homes. Yet, even in the universalist atmosphere of the late 1940s, when it could be assumed that state effort would come to supplant voluntary and charitable provision, Adams (1996: 32) shows that a substantial and enduring role for private welfare was anticipated. It was the 'general assumption' that meals on wheels, for example, 'should be provided through the voluntary sector'. Even mainstream services, such as social work with families 'was provided largely on the assumption that self-help, voluntary effort and help within the family should be sufficient' (Adams 1996: 37).

While the high-water mark of most social policy services had been achieved in the immediate post-war years, the personal social services achieved greatest prominence nearly a quarter of a century later. The term itself was first adopted in the Seebohm Report of 1968, which proposed the creation of unified social services departments within local authorities, providing comprehensive and accessible services for all by whom they might be required. Real expenditure on personal social services, which had remained unchanged during the 1950s, doubled between 1960 and 1968. Direct provision of such services by the state had come, to a greater extent than ever before, to substitute rather than supplement voluntary and charitable action. Yet, below that surface, a 'mixed economy' of private, voluntary and public provision continued to exist and develop. The traditional children's charities, such as Barnardos or the National Children's Homes, adapted their activities to the policies of the new age and survived as suppliers of services in their own right, or as providers of services to local authorities. Changing social needs gave rise to new forms of voluntary organisation, either in the shape of self-help movements or campaigning groups in areas such as disability or mental health. The dominant position achieved by the state in relation to health or education was thus never replicated in the social services.

Moreover, while health and education services were provided free to the user, charging remained an established part of local authority delivery of social services throughout the post-war period. Parker (1976), as quoted by Baldwin (1997: 91), provides a summary of the reasons commonly used to explain and justify this way of working. These include the symbolic value of charging as the expression of an ideological position, regardless of the economic value of any charges levied; the deterrent impact of charges in reducing costs to the taxpayer by reducing demand; the spreading of resources, by reducing the costs of the service while maintaining supply; the reflection of shifting priorities between consumer groups or higher and lower priority services and the prevention of abuse which tying the use of services to a fee was thought to deliver.

In many cases, of course, a decision to charge for services will encompass a combination of these rationales. On the whole, however, as Judge and Matthews (1980: 2) point out, even those administrations opposed to charging in principle, have retained and extended charging when social policy objectives have been subordinated to economic ones. Revenue raising thus dominates the other rationales which have traditionally been offered in justification of charging.

The result of these policy and practice approaches meant that, by 1979, the use of non-state providers and direct charging for services, rendered the social services an area where the acceptance of responsibility by the state and the direct discharge of those responsibilities was less monolithic than in almost all other social policy areas. The marketisation reforms of the 1980s and 1990s, therefore, did not represent a wholly new way of organising such services. While the scale, scope and purpose of privatisation and liberalisation were quite different, the basic mixture of private as well as public effort had never been lost.

The National Health Service

Chapter 8, dealing with the health service, provides a particular concentration upon the development of an internal market and upon the privatisation of capital expenditure through the Private Finance Initiative.

The assumption by the state of universal responsibility for the health of its citizens is essentially a twentieth-century phenomenon. The 1834 Poor Law provided a residual and deterrent service for paupers, through state workhouses. The Victorian contribution in this field was to be found in the profoundly important improvements to collective public health measures of sanitation and safe water supplies. Individuals looking for health care were to make their own provision either directly or through the insurance systems of the trades unions and voluntary societies. The National Insurance Act of 1911 provided the first major alteration in the balance between private and public responsibilities in this area. It introduced compulsory insurance of those earning less than £160 per annum – but not their dependents – in return for guaranteed free access, through an approved society of the subscriber's choice, to the services of a general practitioner and cash payments during periods of sickness. In the view of one contemporary neo-liberal of the privatising Right, it represented one of the 'turning points in the suppression of spontaneous medical provision' (Green 1996: 21). Hospital services were left outside the scope of the 1911 Act and remained, until 1946, the responsibility of the private and voluntary sectors. The effect of the Act at primary care level, however, was considerable. With successive extensions in the groups covered by the Act during the inter-war period, Webster (1988) suggests that by 1938, 43 per cent of the whole population were covered by the scheme.

Whiteside (1998: 205) suggests that the inter-war national insurance arrange-ments displayed many of the characteristics which were later to be claimed as benefits by the neo-liberals of half a century later: Firstly, it was driven by consumer choice; new labour market entrants decided which society to join. Choice was heavily influenced by efficient management; the profitable society offered members better benefits for the same contribution than its less successful competitors. Secondly, as societies competed for new members by providing additional benefits from profits, society rivalry and competition fostered the extension of medical care at no cost to the taxpayer. Despite these advantages, however, the approved society arrangements ended the inter-war period in substantial disrepute. In Whiteside's analysis, three main reasons emerge for this transformation. Firstly, societies were vulnerable to private sector collapse, especially in those areas where industrial depression made greatest demands upon their services. Secondly, private provision involved serious problems of inequity – 'The tendency for the market to provide the best care for those least in need . . . [led to] inverted selection [which] sprang directly from the incent-ive to good management based on values common to any commercial enter-prise.' In other words, those most in need of health care found it most difficult to obtain insurance, and then received the lowest levels of benefit. By contrast, societies assiduously courted the custom of those who were least likely to require their benefits – young, healthy males in full-time employment. Thirdly, the system was condemned for its inefficiency. Competition between suppliers led to duplication of expensive resources, often concentrated in areas where they were least needed. Administratively, industrial assurance companies swallowed up 40 per cent of premium income in such costs. Whiteside (1998: 203) summar-ises the conclusions which were to emerge in the Beveridge Report in this way: 'rationalisation of central surveillance would promote fairness, cost-effectiveness and economies of scale. Competition between service providers caused duplica-tion, waste and high administrative costs; eliminating these effects would secure greater efficiency and fair shares for all.'

The establishment of a universal, free-at-the-point-of-use health service, em-bodying these Beveridgean principles, took place under the 1946 National Health Service Act. This brought hospitals within the scope of public responsibility and extended the scope of primary health coverage to all citizens. The principles of the service are explored in more detail at the start of Chapter 8, but essentially rested upon free and equal access to a service which would provide comprehens-ive treatment on the basis of clinical need, rather than ability to pay. In Bevan's (1978: 109) words, the health service represented, 'a triumphant example of the superiority of collective action and public initiative applied to a segment of society where commercial principles are seen at their worst' *[document 2]*.

Despite this emphatic assertion of public responsibility, however, the debates between private and public provision remained deeper rooted and more per-vasive than might be apparent from the 50-year survival of the National Health Service (NHS) and its enduring place in public affection. From the outset, the principles upon which the NHS was founded were more swiftly under pressure, and that pressure more persistently applied, than its supporters had envisaged. The earliest departure from the basic principle of *free at the point of use* came in the 1949 NHS Amendment Act which introduced charging for prescriptions. In April 1951 Bevan, Harold Wilson and John Freeman famously resigned from the Attlee government over charges for certain dental and ophthalmic services. Rationing, through the waiting list, or what Powell (1996: 33) calls 'the gap between what was medically possible and what was delivered', placed early stresses upon the principle of *comprehensiveness*. Variable levels of services by geography and the continuing gap between the health status of different occupational and social groups soon called into question the achievability, if not the desirability, of the principles of *equality of access and equity of outcome*.

In the years between 1946 and 1997, the Health Service was the subject of a series of official Committees of Inquiry, the first being the 1953 Committee of Inquiry, chaired by the Cambridge economist Claude Guillebaud. At the root of almost all these investigations was alarm at the escalating costs of the service and at the seemingly inexhaustible demand which faced the inevitably finite supply of service. While reports mostly defended the service against accusations of waste and inefficiency – the Guillebaud Report, for example, concluded, as Gladstone (1997: 2) suggests, 'that much of the alarm about the extravagance of the NHS had been misplaced' – the problem showed few signs of resolution. It was against this background that more fundamental critiques of a public health service and a series of alternative solutions, began slowly to emerge. A number of these solutions involved a renegotiation of the responsibilities between public and private spheres with which this book is concerned. Among the strategies to have been attempted before 1979, the more significant included both shifting costs from the collective to the individual and cost cutting through rationing of services.

As already suggested, the principle that cost should be borne by collective rather than individual means was swiftly under pressure in the newly created health service. The general notion that a greater proportion of costs should be recovered from private rather than public sources remained a subject of theoretical debate between the political parties – generally favoured by the Conservatives, generally deprecated by Labour – while in practice, under both parties, although at different paces, moving in this direction. Powell (1996: 33) summarised the situation in relation to prescription charges, the first major departure from the service as originally instituted, in this way: 'In the 1950s the Conservatives extended the charges. Prescription charges were removed by Labour in the 1960s, but quickly returned to become a permanent feature of the NHS landscape.' Revenue-raising strategies, from individual patients rather than taxpayers as a collectivity, continued to preoccupy governments, with recurring attention to the possibility of charging for elements of service such as amenity beds or 'private' rooms.

Attempts by government to cut costs by rationing were developed along two main lines before 1979. Waiting lists for treatment rationed services and thus cut the costs which satisfying that demand would have produced. Increasingly, too, more direct exclusion, by placing certain forms of treatment outside the boundaries of the NHS became a feature of the service. Sometimes there were new advances in medical science which could have provided treatments for hitherto intractable illness or chronic conditions. The heart transplant developments of the 1960s and 1970s, for example, provided one focus around which such discussions surfaced in a relatively public fashion. Other examples involved drawing the boundaries between health services and other 'complementary' forms of treatment more firmly so that osteopaths and chiropractitioners found themselves on one side of the line, while chiropodists and physiotherapists were on the other. The implication was clear. Cost containment within the public system could be achieved by rationing and restricting services within the NHS. Individuals wishing to obtain such treatments would be left to pay directly for the services used. Of course, in redefining the public/private interface in this way, the basic principle that medical need and not cost should determine service provision was placed under severe stress and, in the case of less-well-off individuals, broken. The continuing difficulties led, in 1976, to the setting up, by the Labour government of the latest Royal Commission on the NHS. As Pearson (1992: 217) suggests, its findings were to underpin, 'the Thatcher government's first proposals for NHS reform, in 1979'.

Thus, before the first Thatcher administration took office in 1979, the relationship between public and private provision in health care was already a matter of debate and dispute, both in terms of the scope of services provided and the responsibility for paying for services received. The privatisers and neo-liberals of the 1980s and 1990s were thus part of the longer continuum with which this chapter began and in which the case for diminishing public provision and increasing the scope for private initiative could be developed, not as an unfortunate necessity but as a positive good.

1.2 Using the terms 'privatisation' and 'marketisation'

This chapter now ends by returning to a question posed at the outset: What is the term 'privatisation', as used in this book, intended to convey? It is as well to begin with some warnings. As Hartley (1990: 180) puts it, 'the term privatisation has been the victim of varying definitions embracing deregulation, liberalisation, vouchers, charging for public services previously provided at zero price and the transfer of assets (sales) from the state to the private sector'. Donnison (1984: 107) suggests that the word itself should be 'heavily escorted by inverted commas as a reminder that its meaning is at best uncertain and often tendentious'. Despite the contentious nature of the concept, however, the difficulty of the term lies not only in its tendency to be captured by rival ideological positions but also in the breath of activities which it is used to describe and categorise. Butcher (1995: 108) refers to it as an 'umbrella term' and it is in that broad sense that it is used here, intended to convey a range of techniques through which private, rather than public, activity and responsibility can be increased. It thus encompasses, among others, direct sale of public assets into private hands, the transfer of functions previously carried out directly by the state into the private sector and the withdrawal of the state from responsibilities previously undertaken, leaving such matters to be faced by individual citizens.

Within this latter category, in particular, a key question arises as to whether, as Ranade (1998: 5) asks, 'marketisation and privatisation are conceptually and analytically distinct phenomena'? For Ranade the issue can be resolved by suggesting that the strategies which are part of marketisation 'may lead, as a consequence, to increasing privatisation, if for example, more contracts are won by the private sector in tendering exercises'. While, therefore, 'marketisation and privatisation are not interchangeable concepts . . . in practice, one may lead to the other'. The argument presented in this book is rather different. Privatisation here does not simply refer to a shift of physical goods to the private sector. Nor does it rest at the transfer of responsibilities from public to private – for example, in 'outsourcing' non-clinical services in the NHS – or even in the changing boundary between the public and private purse in meeting the cost of services. Rather, it includes an alteration in the nature of decision making. The creation of markets, rather than single-source providers, results in a widening of those issues over which responsibility has to be exercised, and increases the potential for making different decisions within that wider territory. Within this framework 'choice' has been privatised – removed from the collective public domain, and made the responsibility of private individuals. In that sense, the two concepts are united by a common core: both are concerned with shifting the balance between the public and private spheres, the fundamental issue with which this book is engaged. It is to a more detailed investigation of these questions that Chapter 2 now turns.

Chapter 2

PRIVATISATION

The aim of this chapter is two-fold. Its primary purpose is to trace the history of the privatisation programmes of the 1980s and 1990s, outlining and discussing the ideological and practical considerations by which these initiatives have been shaped and sustained. My intention has been, as far as possible, to provide an account which explores these matters in terms which supporters of the privatisation cause would recognise. In other words, to set out the case upon which privatisation rests. Subsequent chapters will aim to subject this case to scrutiny in the context of specific social welfare services.

2.1 Origins in industrial and economic policy

This book will be concerned with privatisation in the sphere of social policy and social welfare services. Before the thrust towards privatisation in this area began, however, the policy had already been applied – and much celebrated by its authors – in the economic and industrial spheres. Of course, as Vickers and Wright (1989: 3) argue, industrial privatisation, 'raises different questions, involves different actors and policy communities, is motivated by different ambitions, and generates different constraints' from other forms which privatisation has taken. Yet, by the time the Thatcher governments began, in any sustained way, to turn their attention to social welfare services, many of the concerns which had to be addressed, from the technical to the political, had already been rehearsed in the industrial sphere. An investigation of privatisation and marketisation in the social policy field has to be framed, therefore, by some knowledge and understanding of the immediate context from which they were to emerge.

It has often been argued that British privatisation was a policy which was more stumbled upon than set about with deliberate intent (Timmins 1996). A series of writers have emphasised its origins as a pragmatic response to fiscal crisis and its development as shaped more by the pressing need to maximise immediate financial returns than by any ideological commitment to a particular model of private/public relations and responsibilities. Thus, for example, Sir Christopher Foster (1994: 493), senior partner at Coopers & Lybrand, declared categorically that,

'Privatisation would not have happened but for the need to seem to cut public expenditure and borrowing without raising taxation at a time when, as happened throughout the 1980s, there was persistent, but less successful than planned, downwards pressure on public expenditure.'

In the same vein, Marsh and Rhodes (1992: 178) explain the secondary importance accorded to creating competitive conditions in early industrial privatisations in this way:

'the failure to introduce more competition into the initial privatisations of the nationalised industries owed a great deal to the Government's belief that greater competition would reduce the attractiveness of and financial gain from the share issues to small investors and thus the putative electoral advantage to the Conservatives.'

This emphasis upon the fortuitous and the pragmatic, however, was soon eliminated from the Government's own account of its privatisation policies [document 13]. Although privatisation had received no direct mention in the Conservative Party's 1979 election manifesto, by 1983 the Thatcherite Financial Secretary to the Treasury, John Moore, was able to declare that:

Privatisation is a key element in the government's economic strategy. It will lead to a fundamental shift in the balance between the public and private sectors. It is already bringing about a profound change in attitudes within state industries. And it opens up exciting possibilities for the consumer: better pay, conditions and employment opportunities for the employees; and new freedom for the managers of the industries concerned. (As quoted in Bishop and Kay 1988)

A decade later, the Government provided a similarly celebratory definition in response to a United Nations inquiry into comparative experience among member nations. It said:

'The privatisation programme has two main aims: to promote efficiency and to widen and deepen share ownership. Competition is the best way to ensure that goods and services are provided at the lowest economic cost. Giving customers freedom of choice assures sustained pressure on companies to increase efficiency. For employees, privatisation means working in a company with clear objectives, the means to achieve them, and rewards for success. This in turn reinforces concern for the customer.' (Definition presented to the United Nations on 11 May 1993 as reported in United Nations 1995: 3)

2.2 Models of privatisation

Two different models of privatisation seem to jostle for supremacy in this statement. On the one hand, it appears to adopt an approach identified with the Austrian economist, Joseph Schumpeter. The Schumpeterian model emphasises the importance of *private ownership, per se*. The transfer from public to private, through the widened and deepened share ownership, will unleash the forces of enterprise, innovation and entrepreneurial zeal. In this model, the structure of the market is less relevant: be it monopolistic or competitive, the fact of private rather than public ownership will confer the intended benefits.

On the other hand, the Government's definition draws upon a second model which places the emphasis in a different direction. Here, *market conditions* rather than ownership – 'competition is the best way' – are accorded greater importance. In this argument, free, competitive markets confer the benefits of efficiency and the provision of quality services at lowest economic cost. The price mechanism provides the efficient allocation of resources by holding supply and demand in balance. Publicly owned enterprises are capable of delivering such advantages in competitive markets, just as privately owned enterprises are capable of inefficient and expensive services in conditions of monopoly. Indeed, adherents of the more radical right, such as Veljanovski (1987), have dismissed as 'vacuous' the claim that private property is inherently a more efficient form of ownership than public property. Rather than *privatisation*, in the sense of ownership, this second model might more accurately be described as *marketisation*, in its contention that efforts to maximise competition should take precedence over efforts simply to change ownership from public to private.

Linneman and Megbolugbe (1994: 636) suggest that *privatisation* and *marketisation* are best understood as distinct phenomenons. The first is a form of 'load-shedding' in which 'the government divorces itself from both the financing and production of goods and services'. The second is a form of 'empowerment' in which government 'continues to finance public goods and services but leaves their delivery and production to the private sector'. Vickers and Wright (1989: 2), while agreeing that 'there is no logical connection between privatisation and competition', nevertheless suggest that 'it is certainly true that some policies of deregulation have been pursued at the same time as privatisations and have been seen by some observers as intimately linked phenomena'. Letwin (1988), from a position inside the Conservative administrations of the 1980s, claims that it was always the intention of the government that changed ownership and changed market conditions should go hand-in-hand, dismissing suggestions that its advocates 'have not generally claimed that the mere act of privatisation will increase operational efficiency' (Letwin 1988).

The tensions between these rather different approaches to the boundary between state and private activity was apparent in many of the industrial privatisation programmes of the 1980s. Heald (1989) suggests that three distinct phases may be detected in the Thatcher administrations of the period. In the early years, progress was 'relatively modest and exploratory' and limited to returning to private ownership those enterprises which lay at the fringes of government activity. In the middle years, the great public utilities – telecommunications, gas, electricity and water – came under consideration. As monopoly suppliers of essential services, these industries brought to the surface the distinction between ownership and competition outlined above. The shift from the Gas Board to British Gas involved the creation of a private monopoly in place of a public one. It amounted more to a transfer than a transformation. By the time of electricity privatisation, twelve different regional companies were created, paving the way for competition in the future. Nevertheless, at this period, as Heald (1989: 43) suggests, 'when the crunch came, *private ownership* was much higher on the government's priorities than *competition*'.

In the third phase, however, which Heald characterises as 'Finishing the Job', attention turned away from a preoccupation with ownership towards market liberalisation. The shift was pragmatically accomplished, as had been characteristic of the whole privatisation programme, in which, as Heald (1989: 43) suggests, 'to a significant extent, the rationale . . . was invented after the event'. The new emphasis on marketisation and competition was especially directed at the social welfare services which still lay within direct state control, and where the benefits of reform were to be delivered by a combination of privatisation and marketisation techniques.

The complexity of the different forms of government action which fall broadly within the sphere of this book can thus be demonstrated. The central link between privatisation and marketisation, however, lies in the impact which both provide upon the changing division of obligation between the public and private spheres. The period with which we are concerned here is one in which that boundary moved, against the tide of recent history, away from public provision and in favour of private responsibility. A brief discussion of the context within which that shift took place is given below.

2.3 Why was privatisation possible?

Hirschman (1982) has argued that enthusiasm for state or private sector provision operates cyclically, with tides of enthusiasm for one mode rising out of disillusionment with the other. Without following the deterministic conclusions of the Hirschman thesis, it is still possible to detect a strong policy tide which has sustained and extended the reach of the privatisation programme. An increasingly influential school of thought has emphasised the way in which advanced capitalist economies are moving from 'Fordist' to 'post-Fordist' forms of production and consumption. In the Fordist era, the argument suggests, both production and consumption were organised on a mass basis. Post-Fordists argue that the era of large-scale bureaucracies, producing uniform services, is at an end. Hoggett (1991: 247), for example, suggests that we are living in the era of 'post-bureaucratic forms of welfare delivery'. In its place are forms of organisation which emphasise a rapid and flexible responsiveness to customer need, with production individualised to meet the demands of particular groups and individuals. Privatisation then forms part of a set of policies which are wider than itself. At the time when the privatising agenda was at its height, during the middle years of the 1980s and beyond, the strength of the ideological tide in its direction appeared very powerful indeed. Papadakis and Taylor-Gooby (1987: 14), for example, concluded that Britain was in the grip of a 'long-term shift in social ethos away from the collectivism which nourished the welfare state and towards greater valuation of the private in all spheres of social life . . . privatisation of welfare is an idea whose time has come'.

Even when, in terms of public opinion surveys for example, policies were pursued which were not widely supported in advance of their achievement, the constitutional freedom conveyed by the British system played a decisive part in driving them through. Heald (1989: 46) suggests that, 'Political events in the United Kingdom in the 1980s have been shaped by the absence of constitutional protections and the willingness of the Thatcher government to assert centralised power and to override so-called "vested interests".' Of course, in a policy matter there are interests vested both against and for any course of action. The attacks on trade union powers and upon local government are more obviously apparent than the favours afforded to finance capital, newspaper editors and other supporters, but both show a willingness to use the full range of levers of central government power. Indeed, Wright (1994: 6), commenting upon the faster pace at which privatisation proceeded in Britain in comparison with other European states, places emphasis on the 'process of rapid and brutal centralisation' which was the experience in the UK and which, in other countries, was prevented by constitutional arrangements.

Within this realignment of macro-relations, policy networks were also reformulated. In the case of privatisation, as Wright (1994: 26) suggests, this capacity was especially important. Trades unions, local government and even, on occasions, management itself were excluded in order to overcome obstacles in the decision-making process.

2.4 The claimed benefits of privatisation

The claimed benefits of transferring responsibilities from the public to the private sphere include a redefinition of core activities and purposes, together with a reframing of relationships among those most closely involved [document 3]. Within this new framework the dominant modes assume the following roles.

Customers not clients

In this mode the status of the service user is transformed from the weakness of a supplicant, battering at the doors of powerful and unresponsive bureaucracies, to the power of a customer, exercising the rights of choice through paying for services in the market place. In the words of the then-Chancellor of the Exchequer, Sir Geoffrey Howe, in 1981, 'The consumer is sovereign in the private sector. In the public sector he [sic] is dethroned by subsidy and monopoly.' The emphasis upon the sovereignty of the customer depends in turn upon an essentially econometric view of that individual as a competent economic and social actor, capable of making a calculation of her or his own best interests in the market place and following that rational calculation with action. Private entrepreneurs respond, in turn, by a market-oriented motivation in which profit maximisation depends upon attentiveness to the needs of customers seeking quality services and products at lowest prices. Within market theory, as Bowe *et al.* (1993: 26) suggest, 'the aggregate of individual consumer choices is order, equilibrium, a kind of social discipline'. Linneman and Megbolugbe (1994: 637) summarise the interaction in this way: 'Utility-maximising households and profit-maximising firms, if joined by markets covering all desired goods and services, will generally be able to achieve an efficient allocation of social resources.'

As well as changing the status of users, this shift also embraces a realignment of relations between producers of services and consumers in which the primacy of users rather than producers is clearly asserted. Butcher (1995: 139) describes the aim of the market approach in this way:

> 'It argues for greater responsiveness to the public as customers of local services, arguing that local authorities should look at their services from the viewpoint of the public, rather than simply the viewpoint of the local authority. . . . Thus, the public service orientation stresses delivery agencies which are outward looking and proactive, rather than inward looking and reactive.'

Purchasers not providers

In this mode the separation of provision from production allows for a new set of relationships within the design and delivery of social welfare services. As Loughlin and Scott (1997: 205) suggest, 'the welfare state was a service-delivery state, in which government assumed responsibility not only for the provision of a wide range of services but also for their production'. In the new model these functions are separated. Government, in whatever guise, remains responsible for determining the services that are to be provided, but the actual delivery is passed over to separate organisations. In the case of central government, this can be seen, for example, in the separation between the policy-making functions of the Department of Social Security and the implementational responsibilities of the Benefits Agency, as discussed in Chapter 5. In local government, as Chapter 7 sets out, the division may rest between the policy-making or 'enabling' function of Social Services committees and the delivery of these policies by a plethora of organisations in the mixed economy of welfare.

In the shifting boundary between public and private, the separation between commissioning and delivery is sometimes characterised as part of the 'hollowing' of the state, in which central functions are removed or redistributed from the core of public responsibility to a dispersed and disparate Diaspora. The attractions of the separation are apparent to politicians of different persuasions. Deakin and Walsh (1996: 35) summarise the benefits of the policy in this way:

> 'It holds out the promise of a system in which the political agenda can be set at the centre and overall control over implementation retained without acquiring responsibility for tedious detail, so that politicians in power can have the luxury, in the latest cliché, of "steering not rowing".' (Osborne and Gaebler, 1992)

25

Managers not administrators

In this mode, active private sector management methods supplant the more passive public service ethos of public administrators. The ideal of public service is defined by Stewart and Clarke (1987: 167), for example, as one where the emphasis is on 'service *for* the public' and not 'service *to* the public'. The strength of that orientation has, in the view of the New Right, been exaggerated. Public choice theory, upon which the privatisation approach drew heavily, contends that even the most apparently disinterested social welfare professions have disguised or rationalised self-interest as being in the public good. In this way of thinking, the disinterested administrator emerges as a sham against which the claims of management have the advantages of transparency and accountability. The remedy suggested by proponents of the public choice school has been the break-up of large centralised bureaucracies into smaller and competing organisations. In bureaucracies, administrators build empires and are forever protected from the inefficiencies of their own activities. In competing markets, managers reap the rewards and penalties of the decisions for which they can be clearly identified as responsible. The practical effect of this change in social welfare systems can be seen in the transformation of the National Health Service into a large number of independent, local Trusts (see Chapter 8) or the break-up of local education authorities into separate, financially-managed schools (see Chapter 6). Within such new systems, private sector management methods could then be applied. For Ranade (1997: 58ff), the set of techniques thus imported into social welfare systems – accountability mechanisms, performance indicators and reviews, staff appraisal, performance related pay, league tables of performance, quality standards and so on – amount to 'privatisation from within'.

Competition not allocation

In this mode, welfare services such as health and education, rather than being regarded as investment goods which are different in character from other purchases made by individuals, become redefined as consumption goods which may be traded through the supply/demand nexus, as would any other sort of commodity. From the perspective of the reformers, the 'systematic attempts to re-commodify public services' (Kirkpatrick and Lucio 1996: 3) has been part of the effort to increase efficiency and reduce costs. Even more importantly, the market provides an open and transparent means of allocating benefits, rather than the disguised and secretive methods of state bureaucracies. State allocation of goods, supporters of privatisation would argue, makes claims to equity and fairness which cannot be sustained in practice. Rather, 'public' goods become the prerogative of those who are best able to pursue their own interests. Pressure groups, special interest lobbies, well-connected individuals and so on, all operate in a way which seeks to maximise their own benefit, under the cloak of wider public interest. The marketisation of such goods sweeps away these pretences and allows allocation of resources to take place through an open process which maximises beneficial outcomes.

Regulation not planning

In this mode the potential dis-benefits of the market place are contained, not by Fabian-style planning, but by a continued assertion of public interest through the presence of regulation. Possible deficiencies which regulation can make good include circumstances where information necessary to make market exchanges may be incomplete, inaccurate or biased or where an imbalance of information between different players prevents a level playing field. Regulation itself, however, can be organised in a way which remains consistent with redrawing the limits of public action because regulation is delivered by 'arm's-length' organisations, operating with considerable autonomy from Ministers or other politicians. As a result, the obligations and rights of each party have to become more clearly defined, contributing, in the eyes of its supporters, to the additional transparency which privatisation brings.

Moran and Prosser (1994: 3ff), for whom the British privatisation programme represented 'an astonishing achievement', consider it to be 'one of the most important lessons of the privatisation experience in Britain' that 'selling an enterprise to the public sector does not mean an end to questions about public control and accountability. . . . "Privatisation" is not so much a retreat by the State, as a shift in the modes of intervention from ownership to regulation.' Yet, purists of the New Right regard regulation as at best a temporary phenomenon, pending the achievement of truly free markets. In the hands of pluralists and pragmatists, regulation has an importance of its own in relation to equity – a key objective of traditional welfare but one which markets, left to themselves, deliver only weakly. Regulation provides the mechanism by which the efficiency advantages of markets can be retained while ensuring, at the same time, that the interests of the least able actors can be protected and through which unacceptable variation in access or standard of service can be avoided. Some writers, such as Loughlin and Scott (1997: 206) go as far as to suggest that 'the shift towards the regulatory mode of government in the UK may be viewed as a displacement of the welfare state model of government'. Certainly, examples of the shift to hands-off regulation are plentiful, including the industrial examples of Ofwat, Ofgas and Offer (as discussed in more detail in Chapter 3) as well as, in the direct field of social policy, examples such as the creation of Ofsted, the Office for Standards in Education in 1992.

Equality of opportunity not equality of outcome

In this mode, it is claimed, markets provide desert-based equity – that is to say, one where individuals receive fairness because they obtain the results which their own efforts and capacities deserve. The market guarantees that results fairly reflect the relative merits of participants in a contest where each has an equal opportunity of participation but where quality of outcome would be both unachievable and undesirable. Indeed, even when equality of opportunity appears problematic, because individuals begin with different histories and from different contexts, neo-liberal ideology would hesitate to imbue the state with responsibility for amending these inequalities. The defence of fundamental rights of freedom and individual choice is of a higher order than concerns with the distributional or other effects of the market (Miliband 1990: 6).

2.5 Methods of privatisation

An earlier section set out two main models of privatisation. These models have to be translated into practical operation and the different elements which go into that process need to be separated and identified. Wright (1994: 7–8) distinguishes the following components:

- the abolition of or severe curtailment of public services, on the assumption that private provision will fill the gap (seen, for example, in the proliferation of private security firms);
- the squeezing of the financial resources of publicly-funded bodies, in the hope of inducing them to seek compensatory private funding;
- the increase in the financial contribution of consumers for public goods such as medicine;
- the direct transfer to the private sector (often voluntary or charitable) of total policy responsibilities which were previously public;
- the contracting out of public service implementation to private agencies while retaining public responsibility for policy development and commissioning of services;
- the sale of land and publicly-owned housing stock and other tangible assets.

It is immediately apparent, from this list, that 'methods' of privatisation embody within their practicalities some sharply ideological understandings of the state's relationship with individuals and social groups. Their essential continuity rests upon a redrawing of the obligations within that relationship in favour of individual rather than collective responsibility. As Mitchell (1990: 16) suggests, 'perceiving privatisation as the withdrawal of state involvement is both crude and inaccurate'. Rather, actions to transfer assets or to stimulate competition, alter the nature of state involvement rather than eliminate it. The reform of education, for example, included both a very significant strengthening of central power – through the establishment of the National Curriculum – and a transfer of responsibility to school level – in the policy of local financial management. The result, as Hoggett (1996: 17) suggests, is 'the paradox of a public service which has apparently been subject both to more centralisation and decentralisation'.

The benefits which marketisation and privatisation were to deliver in the case of social welfare services thus went far beyond the simple economic. If privatisation began as an economic policy, the advantages which it was to confer in the social sphere lay as much in the liberation of the individual user and the provision of quality services. It is to these claims which this chapter now turns.

2.6 Privatisation and the social welfare services

Wendy Ranade (1997: 20), in her review of health service policy, emphasises the ways in which the general thrust to redraw the boundaries between private and public provision underpinned 'a more specific critique of the state's role in welfare which revolves around two themes: economic efficiency and moral values'. As earlier arguments already explored in this chapter suggest, analysis of privatisation within the social services is an inevitably and inherently ideological enterprise. The assessment and evaluation of moves to increase the role of the private sector and to diminish the public will be different, depending upon the view of such relationships which any individual espouses. Following Salter (1995), the positions given below can briefly be identified as shaping very different ways of understanding or explaining the developments which this book traces.

Fabianism

This is the founding influence upon British social policy thinking and a powerful one still. The rational, planning approach of Fabianism suggests that collective provision would, in the terms of the Beveridge Report, replace the 'inadequate, overlapping, ungenerous and inefficient' character of individualistic welfare systems (Harris 1977: 415). As earlier chapters have shown, the report reacted to the fragmentation and inequalities of post-war social provision and based its arguments for a more collectivist approach on claims which Ranade (1997: 9) has described as 'national efficiency, rationality and the rights of citizenship' and rooted in values of 'equality, equity, efficiency and social integration'. In core parts of the welfare state, services were to be free at the point of use, comprehensive in coverage, available on a universal basis and provided by the state itself. As such they were to have an integrative effect, counteracting the inevitable conflicts produced by capitalism and thus providing a moral as well as an economic advantage. Private provision, by contrast, was more likely to be a 'purveyor of inequality, social division and privilege' (Salter 1995: 18).

Socialism

Socialism is a set of beliefs which are critical of privatisation as an intensification of the social divisions which it holds to be already embodied within the welfare state. The Marxist strand in this perspective, as Ranade (1997: 16) suggests, views the state's involvement in social welfare services in capitalist societies as stemming 'from capital's need to reproduce both labour power and the existing social relations of production which ensures the continued dominance of the bourgeoisie at an economic, political and ideological level'. A number of different radical critiques of welfare provision can also be located within this broad perspective. Feminists, for example, have shown the way in which services which claim to be 'universal' or based on citizenship turn out, on closer examination, to be designed to meet the needs of men not women. Others, from a communitarian tradition, emphasise the need to democratise services, tackle the power of over-mighty professionals and equalise the distribution of services. The user movement has described the institutionalised delivery of welfare as distant, ineffective and alienating in its failure to take seriously the views and experiences of recipients. In the summary provided by Thompson and Hoggett (1996: 27), 'the *general* conception of universalism as procedural impartiality has undermined social diversity through its tendency to confuse impartiality with uniformity and equality of treatment with sameness of treatment'.

Reforms proposed from this perspective emphasise notions of empowerment, rights to welfare and an assault on disadvantage which incorporate an understanding of power and inequality into new forms of diversity and choice. By contrast, privatisation is viewed as a programme which promotes the class interests of capital and privilege, instituted through its political arm, the Conservative Party.

Pluralism

This is a concept in which a mixed economy of welfare, involving both public and private sectors, promotes choice and efficiency, in a trade-off which Evers (1993: 11) describes as 'upgrading rights to risk and diversity at the expense of the traditional emphasis on security and equality'. Pluralists see a positive virtue in variety. A closer balance between public and private provision in welfare is welcomed, not so much because of the intrinsic or superior merits of either, but because from diversity will follow the additional benefits of choice and economy.

Pragmatism

The shift from public to private is argued on the basis that it provides the only way of solving the gap between the public's ever-expanding demand for services, on the one hand, and its diminishing willingness to pay the taxes necessary to fund those services, on the other. Salter (1995: 20) puts it this way:

> 'The history of the welfare state in Britain is the history of the mismatch between demand and supply. Traditionally the imbalance has been handled by a combination of professionally controlled, covert rationing of welfare combined with a gradually expanding tax base which has kept the gap between demand and supply to politically manageable proportions.'

Cutting back on social rights already enjoyed by voters is politically unpalatable; wholesale transfer of provision to an expanded private sector faces difficulties of supply – where would providers of services on this scale be found? Privatisation, through attracting private finance into public welfare, for example, provides a pragmatic compromise in which difficult-to-reconcile policies can continue to be pursued.

Anti-statism and the New Right

This position embraces a set of beliefs which are closest to those which form the central concerns of this book. These include the 'rolling back the state' ambitions of Thatcherism and display the most positive enthusiasm for privatisation from both the Schumpeterian and liberalisation perspectives outlined above. Here the state is viewed as stultifying and inhibiting, undermining personal responsibility and encouraging dependency. From this perspective, the absence of a close and clear connection between the provision of service and its cost also provides perverse incentives for producers to over-provide and consumers to over-consume. The market place, by contrast, fosters the cardinal virtues of self-help and self-reliance (Wright 1994). As Ranade (1997: 20) puts it, 'far from state welfare being a morally superior form of meeting social needs, as claimed by Fabian socialists, for the New Right state welfare is paternalistic and morally bankrupt, rationing resources in a biased and potentially discriminatory way' [documents 3 and 4].

Moreover, from this point of view, the essential claim of the welfare state to be socially integrative makes no sense. 'There is', as Mrs Thatcher so famously remarked, 'no such thing as society.' If there are only individuals and families and a residual, charitable claim to help outsiders, then the whole notion of integrative social welfare services makes no sense. Thus, while pluralists emphasise the opportunity which privatisation provides for increasing diversity and participation, the anti-statists, as Harris (1986: 11) suggests, are far more concerned to use the private and voluntary sectors to substitute for public provision. State welfare, from this perspective, has only a strictly residual role, responsible only for those for whom no other form of essential help can be found.

For the more radical Right, the arguments in favour of the privatisation of social welfare services are thus not simply technocratic or the product of a post-modern disillusionment with communitarian possibilities. The preference for private over public rests upon an unambiguous view of the state as more harmful than helpful. Put briefly, the case includes the following arguments:

- *Economically*, tax-funded services, free to the end-user, disguise true costs and 'gives users incentives to make wasteful use of the services, with the result that use exceeds the level at which the value to users matches the cost to society of providing the services' (United Nations 1995: 186).
- *Morally*, such services create dependency and sap the willingness of individuals to provide responsibly for their own needs and those of their dependants.
- *Practically*, state welfare leads to an ever-growing band of 'rent-seekers', or public sector employees who further their own interests at the expense of service users and those whose taxes pay their wages.

The privatisation of social welfare services, from this perspective, was part of a wider effort to bring new benefits which state provision could not hope to deliver. In the terms used by a United Nations review of comparative privatisation experience, the reforms looked to '*redefine the role of the state* (or rebalance the roles of the public and private sectors) so that the State can concentrate on its core functions, including that of promoting the efficient functioning of markets in the public interest, while leaving the private sector to do what it does best' (United Nations 1995: 4).

2.7 What sorts of competition are possible in social welfare?

Of the two approaches outlined earlier in this chapter, the application of privatisation to social welfare services has drawn less on the direct transfer of assets from public to private – although, as later chapters will demonstrate, this was by no means negligible – than on the attempt to create market conditions in the supply and purchase of services. The process is not a simple one and can take a number of different forms.

From the perspective of privatisation advocates, direct competition within a market place made up of a variety of buyers and sellers, is the preferred option. Even where actual competition to supply services might be only modest the promised benefits could be delivered, provided markets remained open to *contestability*. In this way of thinking, even a market supplied by a monopoly or oligopoly (where a small number of suppliers are dominant) can deliver the benefits of competition, provided, as Ranade (1997: 88) suggests, the possibility exists for new suppliers to 'enter the market relatively easily and inefficient suppliers can be driven out of business'. The threat of competition here is regarded as sufficient to deliver the claimed benefits.

However, if competition within a market is not possible – as can be the case in social welfare conditions – then competition *for* the market on the basis of contracting out and licensing may be an acceptable substitute. It is not surprising, therefore, that the international overview conducted by the United Nations (1995: 182) suggests that,

> '*Contracting out* is the most common option under which community and social services are privatised. The provision of services is contracted out to private enterprises, while the government still retains the responsibility for planning and financing them. The cost of the service and the quality criteria which the private provider is expected to meet are key elements of the service contract.'

Hoggett (1991: 250) suggests that the process involves the abandonment of 'control by hierarchy' – as organised by the traditional welfare state – and its replacement by 'control by contract'. In 1992, the contracting-out approach was further developed by the introduction of the market-testing programme, requiring government departments and agencies to test the cost of providing services themselves against the cost of purchasing them from a private contractor. Chapter 5 will include an examination of these processes in relation to social welfare services.

In the British context, the concept of *quasi-markets* has been developed (most notably by Le Grand) as a way of distinguishing between the sort of market conditions which have been achieved in social welfare services from those in 'true' or 'free' markets. Quasi-market theorists identify a series of ways in which these distinctions may be drawn. Markets in social welfare are not necessarily driven by the profit motive: competition to supply services involves public sector, not-for-profit organisations and private concerns. The culture of competition in quasi-markets is thus more important than the mechanisms and organisational forms through which it is delivered. Nor do purchasers – or customers – within quasi-markets use their own resources: the money continues to be provided by the public purse and through the organisation – local government department or NHS Trust, for example – by which services are required. Purchase is expressed, moreover, as Butcher (1995: 116) suggests, 'in terms of cash, but in the form of an ear-marked sum which can only be used for the purchase of a particular service'. Thus 'customers' in some quasi-markets are rarely individuals themselves; rather, purchase is made on their behalf, by the care-manager or fundholding GP for example, who acts as a surrogate for free-choosing individuals. Implicit in the operation of quasi-markets, however, is the new power of purchasers to press for changes in service provision. Finally, the nature of regulatory systems applied to quasi-markets may be distinguished from those applied in the open market place. A different order of safeguard for the consumer has generally been thought to be required when dealing with social welfare goods such as health or education, as later chapters will demonstrate.

More radical free marketeers prefer *voucher systems*, in which the subsidy is paid not to the supplier – either private or public – but to end-users, who can then purchase services of their own choice using the monetary value of the voucher to cover all or part of the costs incurred. In the British experience, to date, voucher systems have enjoyed only limited and experimental use. In the field of education, however, as Chapter 6 demonstrates, a theoretical preference for the approach has displayed a considerable vitality and at least one practical application of some significance.

Whatever form of marketisation may be preferred, however, the application of such techniques to social welfare were intended, as Deakin (1996: 21) suggests, to make available 'the crucial virtues of the market, as presented by its advocates: clarity of purpose and allocation of responsibilities, simplicity in operation, and working with the grain of motivation in tapping entrepreneurial and competitive instincts and harnessing them to quality in service delivery'.

2.8 Summary

This chapter now ends with a brief summary of the main advantages which have been claimed for the privatising and marketising measures of the past twenty years and an indication of the ways in which these claims will be tested against their practical application in the series of policy contexts which form the subject of the chapters which follow.

The New Right preference for private rather than public forms of provision rests upon a series of key claims, capable of being applied in different combinations. This chapter has highlighted six main reasons for advancing private rather than public solutions to social policy questions. These may be summarised as follows:

1. The inherent advantages of private over public ownership. In the government's own definition, 'The transfer from public to private, through the widened and deepened share ownership, will unleash the forces of enterprise, innovation and entrepreneurial zeal.'
2. The importance of marketisation and competition which privatisation provides: 'Competition is the best way to ensure that goods and services are provided at the lowest economic cost. Giving customers freedom of choice assures sustained pressure on companies to increase efficiency.'
3. The advantage of transparency, in which real prices can be attached to services provided, thus fostering their responsible use by consumers and their economical provision by suppliers.
4. The benefits of a realignment of core relationships in which the interests of customers or purchasers, rather than providers or suppliers are paramount. The weak base of citizenship claims upon services are thus supplanted by the more powerful and real claims which customers are able to assert in the market place.
5. The introduction of new management techniques into formerly public sector administrations, supplanting large, bloated, protected, inefficient and self-seeking bureaucracies with lean, mean, accountable and efficient enterprises, earning their rewards and fulfilling their obligations to accountability by satisfying customers in relation to quality and price of services.
6. Through the 'rolling back the state' come a further set of advantages in the reformulation of relationships between the individual citizen and the state. The moral bankruptcy of an all-embracing state, undermining personal responsibility and encouraging dependency will be replaced by the morally and economically preferable virtues of self-help and self-reliance. The substitution of private for public thus provides not only increased diversity and participation but also, and more importantly, an intrinsic and moral advantage in a more honest set of relationships between citizen and state.

As suggested at the start of this chapter, these ideas were first developed and applied within industrial, rather than social policy agendas. The claims made by the privatisers and free marketeers now need to be tested against their practical application. Chapter 3 begins this process by investigating an area where economic, industrial and social policy interests overlap – the privatisation of the great utility companies of gas, water and electricity.

Chapter 3

PRIVATISATION, THE UTILITIES AND SOCIAL POLICY

The previous chapter set out a series of claims which advocates of privatisation have made on its behalf. This chapter aims to subject the cited advantages to a first test, in order to provide a fuller framework within which the application of privatisation and marketisation to social welfare services may be scrutinised and assessed. The testing ground will be the operation of the privatised utilities of gas, water and electricity. A three-fold rationale underpins this decision.

Firstly, an exploration of the claims of privatisation in relation to the utilities provides a context in which the New Right project can be assessed in its own terms. Nowhere have the advantages of shifting responsibility from public to private been more loudly or unambiguously proclaimed than in relation to these industries.

Secondly, while privatisation of the utilities has generally been presented and debated in economic terms, the shift from public to private in these industries has produced a set of social policy consequences which, once identified and assessed, will provide material of considerable significance in the investigation of social welfare services themselves.

Thirdly, the industries provide a relatively transparent means of tracing the impact of privatisation upon poorest customers. Equity is a core claim of the welfare state and will form an essential element in the consideration set out in later chapters of the impact of privatisation upon social welfare services. The record of privatised utilities in relation to poorest consumers will provide an illuminating context within which the key issues can be identified and explored.

The chapter begins with a consideration of the benefits which privatisation in this field can be said to have delivered, assessing the ways in which these benefits have been distributed among significant stakeholders in the industries. This section tests some of the central claims of privatisation, including the broadening of the base of stakeholding, through the creation of a 'shareholding democracy', and, through the operation of market mechanisms, to have spread its benefits more efficiently and equitably than a publicly-run and delivered service. A small case study from within the electricity industry will consider the relative fates of shareholders, directors and workers in a liberalised market. It ends with a suggestion that the economic successes of privatisation may have more hidden social costs which do not fall to the companies themselves.

The second section focuses in more detail upon the way in which the operation of the privatised utilities has had an effect upon customers, and upon poorest customers in particular. It begins by looking at some key policy developments in the industries, which revolve around central claims for the benefits of privatisation: competition and innovation.

The chapter ends with a third section which considers the role of the regulator in the privatised utilities and, particularly, looking at the claims which Chapter 2 outlined, in relation to the role of regulators in promoting equity in market outcomes.

3.1 Privatisation and the utilities

The privatisation of the utilities fits squarely into a number of the categories identified in Chapter 2. The shifting of these industries from public to private represented the high-water mark of Thatcherism, occurring after the more tentative approaches of the 1979 administration and leaving only the further fringes of the public sector to be tackled in the 1990s *[document 4]*. The form of privatisation was straightforward too. Other than the sale of council housing (as discussed in Chapter 4), it represented the greatest direct transfer of ownership from public to private hands of all the privatisation programmes. In the place of ownership, the protection of public interest was to be provided through arm's-length regulation, set up through the new great Offices of Regulation for Gas (Ofgas), Electricity (Offer) and Water (Ofwat).

The gas industry was the first to be privatised in 1986. It represented the most complete transfer of a public monopoly into a monopoly in private hands. In many significant ways British Gas plc differed little from its state-run predecessor. For its 18 million domestic consumers it remained, for a further ten years, a monopoly supplier offering neither choice nor diversity.

The water industry in England and Wales was privatised in 1989. In Scotland and Northern Ireland the industry remains in public hands. The most important tasks of the industry were identified by the National Consumer Council (1994) as the provision of a commodity, 'essential to everyday living and supplied on a monopoly basis'. There are approximately 20 million domestic consumers of the privatised water companies.

The electricity industry was privatised in 1990 with 12 Regional Electricity Companies (RECs) made responsible for the distribution and supply of electricity to some 22 million individual consumers in England and Wales. It was, according to Ernst (1994), the 'most complex and troublesome' of all the privatisations. The subsequent history has been one of mergers, take-overs and, beginning in September 1998, the first moves to competition in the domestic supply market.

The case for privatisation of the utilities rested firmly on the core claims set out in Chapter 2. Private ownership would bring the inherent advantages of enterprise and efficiency. Real democracy would be extended to the industries through share ownership and the powerful claims which customers are able to assert in the market place. The management skills of the private sector would be applied in the place of public sector administration, transforming large, bloated, protected, inefficient and self-seeking bureaucracies into lean, mean, accountable and efficient enterprises, earning their rewards and fulfilling their obligations to accountability by satisfying customers in relation to quality and price of services. The 'rolling back the state' was to produce a further set of advantages in the reformulation of relationships between the individual citizen and the state. The moral bankruptcy of an all-embracing state, undermining personal responsibility and encouraging dependency, was to be replaced by the morally and economically preferable virtues of self-help and self-reliance. The substitution of private for public thus provided not only increased diversity and participation but also, and more importantly, an intrinsic and moral advantage in a more honest set of relationships between citizen and state.

Implicit in all utility privatisations, and inherent in the claims which the policy makes to transparency and honesty, economy and efficiency, lies the translation of public goods-for-use into private goods-for-sale. 'Commodification', as Chapter 2 explained, places water, gas and electricity in the market place on a par with any other goods, to be bought and sold between self-interest maximising consumers and profit-maximising producers. Clarity and equity would be the result.

Profits

The first claim of privatisation was that private ownership, *per se*, would bring with it the advantages of enterprise and innovation. If profitability is used to test this claim then, as Graham (1997) suggests, 'The UK utility sector is one of the most lucrative industries in the country. Profits for all utilities reached £7.7 billion in the financial year 1994/95.' Since the onset of privatisation, the companies involved have between them generated total profits of over £60 billion (*Labour Research* 1997b). The generating companies in the privatised electricity industry, for example, National Power, PowerGen and the National Grid Company have between them produced profits of over £4 billion since their respective sell-offs, placing them among the top fifty profit makers in Britain.

Advocates of privatisation, however, do not rest their claims upon profitability *per se*. Through the operation of market mechanisms, the advantages of privatisation were to be spread more efficiently and equitably than had been possible under the old nationalised, publicly-owned and run system. The benefits of efficiency and entreprenerialism were to have been felt by all those involved in the industries – shareholders, managers, workers and customers. The following sections consider how far these claims stand up to actual performance.

Stakeholders

Shareholders

There can be little doubt that profitability in the privatised utilities has been turned decisively to the benefit of shareholders. In the case of British Gas, total dividends rose by 269 per cent between 1987 and 1992. In the water industry, where rising profits took place at the same time as prices to consumers rose sharply, shareholders witnessed an average growth in dividend payments of 63 per cent a year between 1989/90 and 1992/93 (National Consumer Council 1994: 24/49). In the first year of privatisation, earnings per share within the privatised electricity companies increased by 58 per cent.

Yet, if shareholders have prospered, the much-vaunted 'shareholding democracy' which formed one of the main claims of privatisation has fared less well. The pattern which emerged in each of the industries was one in which large numbers of early shareholders soon left the market. The sale of the Regional Electricity Companies at the end of 1990, for example, created around 9 million electricity shareholders. Within six months, 60 per cent of shareholders had cashed in their holdings. Currently there are some 2.5 million. In the case of British Gas there were 4.5 million successful applicants for shares in December 1986. This number had fallen to 2 million by 1988. There were 1.8 million in mid-1995. The ten water and sewerage companies were privatised in December 1989. Within six months the total number of shareholders had fallen by half to 1.3 million and has since fallen by a further 400,000.

Nor are these figures simply the result of individual shareholders making decisions of their own volition. In the wake of the disquiet displayed by large numbers of shareholders in the 'fat cat' remuneration scandals of 1995, some of the privatised companies have made it plain that they regard the small shareholder as a nuisance. Early in 1996, British Gas chair Richard Giordano showed a waning enthusiasm for popular capitalism when he said he wanted to reduce the number of small shareholders in the company. As he put it: 'We have to find a way to ease Aunt Maud out without any pain.'

The declining number of small shareholders is significant because it casts doubt upon some of the key claims of the privatisers: democratisation and diversification are the benefits which widespread shareholding was intended to deliver. The history of the privatised utilities does not suggest that these have been successfully achieved. Moreover, the decline of small shareholdings alters the balance of advantage between different stakeholders in the privatisation settlement. Shareholders who cease to hold shares remain potential stakeholders as possible employees, customers and citizens. This section now turns to one such remaining category, that of directors and senior managers.

Managers

The importation of private sector management methods into previously public organisations is a consistent and much-emphasised advantage claimed by supporters of privatisation. Yet, the history of management in the privatised utilities has not been a happy one. The image of the privatised gas industry suffered badly from its decision, in November 1994, to award its Chief Executive, Cedric Brown, a 75 per cent pay increase. His salary level of £475,000 sparked off the start of the 'fat cat' pay rows which have since continued to be a feature of all the privatised utilities. Problems have also occurred in relation to transparency and accountability, two of the key benefits which new management approaches were said to deliver. In addition to direct remuneration, investigation of accounts at Companies House in Cardiff have revealed the extent to which company directors have benefited directly from the take-overs and mergers which have become rife in the privatised utilities. The money paid in these circumstances is hidden. It has none of the glare of publicity which has surrounded the direct payments which companies make to their executives. During the take-over boom of 1995 and 1996, however, £27 million was given in this way to company directors in compensation for loss of office, top-up pension contributions, share options and last minute pay rises.

Workers

In turning to consider the impact of privatisation upon workers in the gas, water and electricity industries this chapter deals, for the first time, with a group for whom its consequences have been less advantageous. Since privatisation, the scale of job losses in the three industries has been formidable. As advocates of privatisation would have predicted, the impact of private ownership and the use of private sector management techniques have led to extensive 'efficiency gains' and large-scale 'shake-outs' from over-manned enterprises. The success, in 1995, of Scottish Power's hostile bid for the regional electricity company, Manweb, for example – which entailed paying nearly 30 per cent more than the stock market had valued the company on the Friday evening before the bid was launched – was to be financed, according to industry analysts, by the transfer to Manweb of Scottish Power's more efficient management methods.

In what way were the costs and benefits from this operation of the privatised market distributed?

Shareholders are the key to any take-over and their support had been expensively bought. By the time a majority had been convinced to transfer their loyalty to Scottish Power, the price of their conversion was an offer of 975p for each of their shares. At privatisation the same items had been sold at 240p each.

As to directors, several of the Manweb directors, who had attempted unsuccessfully to resist the take-over, resigned at the end of the month, taking with them £1.3 million in compensation for loss of office and a further £1 million in other benefits such as enhanced pension contributions.

It was upon Manweb workers that the costs of the take-over were to fall most directly because, in the context of industry take-overs, the 'more efficient methods' through which the benefits to shareholders and directors were to be financed, can be construed more simply as job losses. When the Scottish Power bid was launched, Manweb employed some 4,500 workers, compared to 5,500 at privatisation. In September 1994 it had announced plans to shed 500 of its 4,500 staff. Together with the company's existing severance scheme, this envisaged staff members being reduced to around 3,000 by 1996. Scottish Power's plans depended on being able to reduce this number significantly further. As Will Hutton suggested:

> '[Scottish] will need to squeeze cost savings of a good £30 to £40 million a year from Manweb's operations in order to service that extra £300 million of debt and shares. The bulk of Manweb's costs are buying electricity from the pool to pass on to customers: these costs are fixed. There is a £100 million wage bill to be attacked – this is what the "neutral" language over costs means. If the headquarters at Chester is not closed it will be reduced to a husk; there will be lay-offs and wage reductions; and some deterioration in the service that Manweb customers receive. No other way of making savings exists. . . . Customers and workers, two key stakeholders in this monopoly, are cast as spectators in the process – even while their interests are being neglected.' (*The Guardian* 25.7.95)

The costs of utility job losses was analysed in a report from the industry union, Unison. It showed that, since privatisation in 1990, staff levels in the electricity industry had fallen from 144,219 to 102,197. The 10,000 jobs shed between March 1994 and March 1995 alone were estimated to have cost taxpayers £40 million in lost tax and benefit payments.

The leading American regulator, Gregory Palast, has suggested that Britain never experienced privatisation in a true free-market sense. Rather, he suggests, the shift of the utilities from public to private represented a privatisation of profit, but a socialisation of risk. In this analysis, the companies retain all the economic advantages which inevitably accrue to monopoly suppliers of essential goods, while the social costs of their actions fall to others. Thus, as water companies shed labour, their failure to tackle leaking pipes creates costs in environmental detriment and failing service to the public. The financial costs of redundancy, in the meantime, are borne by the public sector in terms of benefit claims, taxes forgone, as well as less direct costs in terms of ill-health, skill depletion and so on.

Customers

The claims to innovation, efficiency and enterprise which are at the heart of the privatisation agenda thus need some qualification in practice. The single greatest caveat which has to be applied lies in relation to the claim that privatisation was a strategy from which *all would benefit*. The doubts raised in relation to the very different outcomes for shareholders, executives and workers appear all the more acutely in relation to the case of customers, to which this chapter now turns. In the case of Manweb and Scottish Power, for example, while workers were to carry the immediate costs of restructuring, customers were also placed outside the circle of beneficiaries. Scottish Power made it clear that customers were not to expect any immediate share in the financial advantages upon which their bid for Manweb had laid great weight. Indeed, their plans showed that it would be at least four years before any of the benefits of changed ownership might trickle down to customer level. Moreover, in their guise as taxpayers, the same customers would have to take their share of the public costs which the actions of private companies had produced. In the next sections of this chapter, attention will be directed towards two areas in which the case for privatisation has been particularly strongly made: the benefits of competition, together with its allied phenomenon of cost-reflective pricing, and the advantages of innovation and entrepreneurial flair.

Markets

Competition

In its initial stages, the privatisation of utilities fell very clearly within the Schumpeterian model in which the transfer of ownership *per se*, from public to private, was intended to provide new and substantial benefits. The intention to create a competitive market gained force as an ambition, however, as the programme developed. The ability of customers to choose from a range of different suppliers in competition with one another was portrayed as a more-or-less unalloyed good, in which prices would be kept down and services improved through the operation of the market. This view was largely shared by both industry regulators and Customer Services Committees. In practice, however, competition is less straightforward. As Baker (1997) suggests, 'the transition from monopolistic supply to free markets, however, is highly complex and can easily reinforce existing distortions in supply and consumption. Low income consumers almost inevitably fall further behind during the process of transition.'

By September 1999 the domestic market for both gas and electricity will be fully operational and, in the case of gas, will have experience extending over three years, since the first introduction of competition in the South West of England in April 1996. The major independent scrutiny of developments in the gas industry in the South West is that reported by Waddhams-Price (1997: 121). She makes clear the very particular context within which the pilot introduction of domestic competition took place: 'Many players have a vested interest in seeing competition succeed: the government, the regulator and the new entrants will all try to make the early phases "appear good" because so much hangs on the outcome for the entire residential market for energy to be liberalised in 1998.' Despite these 'good behaviour' incentives, the results were disquieting. It soon emerged that, in a competitive market, while some customers are unwanted, others are assiduously courted; there are those whom existing companies wish to keep and those whom they do not strive officiously to retain. Unwanted customers are those who contribute least to the profits of the new supply companies. Indeed, the evidence from the South West strongly suggests that competition leaves poorest customers worse off. Companies inevitably make greatest efforts to sign up the customers whom they find most attractive, and do so primarily by differential pricing.

Guy *et al.* (1997: 210) cite the following example from the South West experience:

'An affluent gas consumer, subject to cherry-picking and able to pay by direct debit, could obtain competitive gas supplied from Calor Tex for 36 pence per therm. A marginal customer, on the other hand, unable to tempt in new competitors, would be trapped as a customer of British Gas, forced to use a prepayment meter, and be charged 81 pence per therm.'

In Professor Waddhams-Price's conclusion, these regressive changes – in which poorest consumers pay more, and well-off customers pay less – are *'an inevitable consequence* of introducing competition' (emphasis added). The upshot is that

'the most vulnerable consumers are in danger not only of being excluded from the benefits of competition, but of footing the bill for the introduction of benefits which others will enjoy'. As well as morally offensive, the economic consequences of such changes are, as she further notes, 'particularly worrying when other safety nets are simultaneously being weakened'.

Cost-reflective pricing

The essential mechanism through which competition alters the balance of prices between different groups of customers is cost-reflective pricing. At the time of nationalisation, a requirement had been placed upon the utilities 'not to show undue preference towards or discrimination against any consumer or group of consumers'. This was generally interpreted by them as requiring that no distinction be made in prices charged, regardless of the location of consumers or the way in which they paid their bills, even where the company incurred different costs (Waddhams-Price 1997). This understanding has been entirely reversed on privatisation, since when 'undue discrimination' has been interpreted as prohibiting the cross-subsidisation of any one group of consumers by another. To give just one example, the electricity industry has consistently passed on to its poorest customers the cost of providing them with prepayment meters. The South Wales company, SWALEC, for example, charges its prepayment customers an extra £32.20 on the basis that the meter itself produces such costs in installation and upkeep. As Marvin and Guy (1997: 123) put it,

'pre-privatisation, nationalised utilities provided uniform services based on average cost pricing and a universal quality of service. However, with privatisation, utilities are now facing increasing competition and are under severe commercial pressure to differentiate services by price, quality, and time of use to different types of customer, in order to raise profits through heightened operational efficiency. This means replacing cross-subsidies from large to small customers with a new emphasis on real-time, cost-based pricing.'

To summarise: privatisation lays great claims upon the benefits which competition would bring – benefits which were to be available to all classes of consumer. The operation of the market, however, in the privatised utilities has not seen this contention borne out in practice. Rather, it shows considerable signs of conferring its benefits upon those who, in social policy terms, could be said to need them the least, while heaping new costs upon those least able to bear them. Cost-reflective pricing suggests that this is not an unintended consequence of competition: rather it is inherent, intrinsic and inevitable when market conditions are allowed to operate in relative freedom. Not all supporters of privatisation claim that its advantages would be equally distributed among the whole population. Even those who expect a differential distribution, however, generally claim that everyone will end up better off than before. The accumulating evidence of marketisation in the utilities suggests that this is unlikely and that, rather, some groups and individuals will be absolutely worse off as a result of the changes. This chapter now considers the ways in which such a set of changes impacts upon the division of responsibility between the public and the private sphere, concentrating upon an example rooted in the innovation and entrepreneurial flair which advocates of privatisation cite as one of the main benefits of reform. The example is that of new technology and prepayment metering.

Technology and prepayment metering

While cost-reflective pricing may have been driven by commercial considerations, it has been made possible by a revolution in the technology available to the privatised industries. As Graham (1997: 143) points out, the effect of new technology is to allow 'highly individualistic private-market solutions to be imposed over what were previously quasi-public goods'. In the case of the utilities, prepayment metering – in which consumers have to pay in advance through tokens or rechargeable keys – is a method which has come to dominate the provision of these essential services to the poorest citizens and whole disadvantaged communities. In the process it has allowed companies a particularly advantageous method of disengagement from the unprofitable and problematic part of their market, relocating responsibility for access to such basic services firmly with poorest customers themselves. These changes have spatial as well as individual consequences, with both those most affected, and the effects themselves, concentrated in particular geographical locations. For the purposes of this chapter, these developments will be reviewed primarily through investigation of the performance of the privatised water companies.

3.2 Poorest customers and privatisation

Debt and disconnection have, from the outset, been a constant source of concern to the privatised companies. In 1995, Herbert and Kempson had established that while, in 1989, fewer than 1 per cent of households had fallen into arrears on water bills, by 1994 this figure had grown to 9 per cent, or almost 2 million households. By 1997 Graham was reporting a recent survey in which it was found that, '75% of people on Income Support . . . now have difficulty paying water bills, and that problems of water debt are rising faster than any other form of debt'.

Sharply rising water prices, in the years immediately following privatisation, were accompanied by a rapid rise in disconnection figures. Public disquiet followed and, under pressure from the regulator, the industry looked to solutions which had already been developed in gas and electricity where disconnections had fallen sharply since privatisation. The Welsh company, Dwr Cymru, for example, embarked upon a rapid programme of prepayment metering in the early months of 1994. Between April of that year and January 1995 the number of units in use had risen from 328 to 1,995. In July 1995 it had grown to 2,400. Within eighteen months the figure had shown a further seven-fold increase, to 17,800 units. Prepayment devices had already come to outstrip long-established payment methods such as fortnightly payment cards and was due to overtake direct payment from benefit as the most likely payment method for those in significant debt. By the time such devices were declared illegal by the High Court in February 1998 (see below) the number of prepayment units installed by the company was close to 30,000.

Prepayment use in the water industry illustrates the rapid growth of such devices in the privatised utilities as a whole. The earlier start upon prepayment metering in gas and electricity had led, by September 1997 to 1,107,816 gas customers and 3,690,000 electricity customers purchasing a supply in this way (Houghton *et al.* 1998). As has been argued elsewhere (Drakeford 1997a), the shift to prepayment provides significant advantages for companies, including the collection of revenue in advance of consumption, a secure way of recovering debt while avoiding the costly procedures of Court action or the employment of recovery agents and leapfrogging over other creditors.

For customers, however, prepayment gives rise to a series of practical difficulties – availability of outlets, opening hours, denominations in which tokens are available or keys may be recharged – (see, for example, Rowlingson and Kempson 1993; Sheffield Business School 1994; Drakeford 1995). These difficulties add to the direct and opportunity costs – mechanical problems, loss of cards and higher tariffs – involved in relying upon such devices. The need to visit an outside location in order to activate a service network available within the home has been described as the modern equivalent of pre-industrial social organisation (Graham 1997). In the water industry, for example, the key-charging or token-selling points are the equivalent of wells which individuals have to visit in order to obtain a supply. An analysis of such prepayment customers, conducted for the Gas Consumer Council in 1997, revealed them to be young (with over 37 per cent aged 18 to 30 compared to only 5 per cent over 65), poor (with 40 per cent having household incomes of less than £5,000 per annum and 76 per cent less than £15,000) and struggling (with 35 per cent described as 'just about surviving', and living in areas of very low incomes and high unemployment). Unsurprisingly, most say they have prepayment meters to pay back debts (36 per cent), to budget (22 per cent) or a combination of both (18 per cent). A large majority (84 per cent) also had an electricity prepayment meter fitted. A similar picture of prepayment issues arises in the electricity industry where a further 300,000 prepayment meters in debt cases were installed in 1996/97.

The most significant difficulty associated with the use of prepayment meters, however, lies in the impact they have upon the ability to gain access to a minimum necessary supply of these most basic services. Even for those who are not cut-off (see below), prepayment devices have the effect of reducing consumption beyond a level which is consistent with health, safety and participation in the normal patterns of community life. The *Hidden Disconnected* study carried out by the Birmingham Settlement in 1992 found that the introduction of prepayment meters had a dramatic effect in reducing fuel consumption in the households interviewed. This was achieved by, for instance, cutting the number of cooked meals and minimising the use of hot water. Moreover, despite and following all such efforts to maintain a supply, all those interviewed had experienced periods of energy deprivation or 'self-disconnection'.

The phenomenon of *self-disconnection* occurs when those relying upon prepayment meters fail to buy tokens or recharge keys. The supply of gas, electricity and – in a different fashion – water then comes to an end. The scale of self-disconnection from the privatised utilities has been investigated in a series of research projects. A MORI survey (MORI 1995) conducted for the water industry showed that between March 1993 and July 1994, 80 per cent of households with a prepayment device used the emergency credit facility and 10 per cent had their water supply 'shut off' completely for more than 24 hours because they had not recharged their water keys. Notifications to local environmental health officers in the same area suggest that 273 of the 1,027 households with prepayment devices had gone without water for 24 hours or more. Figures from one company's own trials – Severn Trent – suggested that 49 per cent of customers in the trial had been without a water supply after running out of emergency credit (National Local Government Forum Against Poverty 1995). Of those cut off for more than seven hours, 28 per cent borrowed water, 18 per cent stored water with the attendant public health risks, while 13 per cent went without water altogether. By 1996 the journal, *Utility Week*, reported that two-thirds of households using water prepayment meters experienced 'self-disconnection' during the first year in use. A report produced by the Centre for Sustainable Energy (Houghton *et al.* 1998: 20) suggested that, if the rate of self-disconnection from electricity and gas uncovered in its survey were to be repeated nationwide, 'it would be the equivalent of one million households going without'.

3.3 The regulator

Prepayment meters have produced a parallel fall in the number of customers whom the privatised utilities have cut off from a supply of essential services. In doing so, they have allowed companies to avoid the public opprobrium which accompanied the contrast between highly rewarded shareholders and directors on the one hand, and the treatment of poorest customers on the other. In the process, however, public disconnection has been replaced, rather than eliminated, by the private processes of self-disconnection. A brief codicil to this account needs to consider the role of the regulator, the system which, as Chapter 2 discussed, is intended, within the privatisation programme, to compensate for any deficiencies which an unrestrained market system might produce. Once again, the water industry provides the most instructive example.

In the autumn of 1995 a consortium of local authorities, anxious about the public health and other consequences of self-disconnection through water pre-payment meters, attempted to persuade the Office of Water Regulation to declare the installation of such devices illegal. The authorities relied upon legal advice that prepayment meters which resulted in being cut off from a water supply contravened the requirements of the Act which brought the privatisation of the water industry into being. That Act included, as a result of lobbying at the parliamentary stages, a set of protections for individuals under threat of disconnection which, the local authorities argued, prepayment meters allowed the companies to circumvent. The Director General of Ofwat, Ian Byatt, dis-agreed. In June 1995, he published a circular letter to all managing directors of water companies in England and Wales (Ofwat 1995), which signalled the clear support of the regulator for the prepayment system. Dealing with legal ques-tions which had been raised about the method, the regulator lined up firmly with those who argued that a system which allowed 'self-disconnection' – because of inability to pay – did not amount to disconnection by the supplier: it was the customer, not the company, who was exercising the choice to go without water.

Faced with this decision, the local authorities decided to seek a judicial review of the regulator's decision. In February 1998, Mr Justice Harrison, at the High Court, granted the declaration sought by the local authorities, deter-mining that the cutting off of water by a Budget Payment Unit (the preferred term within the industry itself) amounted to a breach of the companies' duties under the Act and of the statutory code of practice by which their actions in relation to poorest customers, in particular, is regulated. The authorities had submitted five separate issues for determination and were successful in all cases. The Judge concluded that it was 'common-sense' that disconnection had taken place in circumstances where the prepayment meters shut down the water supply. The argument that this was the responsibility of the customer, not the company, was 'superficially attractive but not logically correct'. The operation of the devices did not, as the regulator contended, represent only a 'trivial' violation of the Act. Nor did the law allow the Director General, as he claimed, to refrain from action if he considers that BPUs, although unlawful, are in the best interests of some customers.

So it was that, far from operating in such a way as to mitigate the excesses of the market place, the regulatory system in the water industry was found to have acted in direct contravention of the law and against the interests of the group of customers most in need of the protection of regulation. Even the law, however, has proved to be an uncertain source of help in the face of the powerful new privatised utilities. Following the High Court judgement the Director General of Ofwat wrote to the managing directors of all water companies. This letter made it clear that the continued capacity of BPUs to cause disconnection in any circumstances – consumers subject to county court judgements, partial or limited flow solutions and so on – had been found unlawful and should be brought to an immediate end. Six months later, however, Welsh Water, the company with the largest number of devices, had failed to make public even its plans for the removal of devices which it had installed with such alacrity. Rather, it had embarked upon a policy of adjusting the prepayment meters only being opened 'where requested' by the consumer and proposed, in future, to install reduced flow valves to replace the disconnection mechanism. In such cases, individuals who failed to buy tokens for a prepayment meter could be allowed a radically reduced flow of water so as to allow, over time, for such basic necessities, such as filling a kettle or flushing a toilet to be accomplished. Such devices – known in the field as 'trickle-flow' – had been expressly addressed in the letter sent to water companies by the regulator in response to the High Court judgement. In the final paragraph of that letter, Mr Byatt had made it plain that, while some companies were known to be interested in the development of a reduced flow system, 'its application would be inconsistent with the Judgement and would require amending legislation'. Despite this unequivocal advice, Welsh Water embarked upon 'a managed roll out of replacing existing valves with the new reduced flow valve, this will be a mix of new and existing customers'. Not only was this circumvention of the order obtained from the Court to be applied to the 28,144 customers who by now had prepayment devices installed, but to the 1,779 new customers waiting to be drawn into the scheme.

The response of Welsh Water to the High Court decision casts considerable light upon a further key claim of the privatisers – that accountability would be strengthened in the new system. Customers, using their power in the market place, were to exercise a direct influence over providers which had not been possible in the status as citizen-owners of nationalised companies. Where raw market forces needed taming, in order to fulfil social obligations, regulation, drawing on the full force of the law would ensure that action followed. In fact, as demonstrated here, not only do some customers have very little power in the market place, but even when, and in the teeth of regulatory opposition, they are able to mobilise the law on their behalf, the response to legal direction is further differentiated by power and access to resources. When poor people fail to pay their bills, neither the companies nor the regulator display any hesitation in declaring that the full range of penalties should be available in order to ensure that they are required to meet their obligations. How differently matters are negotiated when a company finds itself at odds with its obligations. Welsh Water, faced with a judgement which it did not favour, has been able to obtain legal advice of its own which has enabled it to act in a way which, in the view of those by whom the judgement had been obtained, violates its intentions. It has been able to do so without the consent, or even the direct knowledge, of the Regulator. Only sustained pressure by individuals, campaigning groups and media interest finally produced an admission from the Regulator that Welsh Water were acting in defiance of the law and a renewed instruction issued to the company to alter its intentions. Almost a year had now elapsed since the

High Court ruling. While the regulator denied that the events of the interven-
ing period had suggested any deficiency in the power of his office, or his willingness to deploy those powers, poorest customers in Wales remained without the
protections which privatisation had promised.

3.4 Summary

Privatisation of the basic utility industries in England and Wales has thus produced a settlement in which advantages have shifted significantly towards those
least in need of them, while disadvantages accrue to those who find them most
difficult to sustain. The claims of efficiency and entrepreneurialism turn out to
have been achieved at very considerable cost to equity. Market relations, far
from providing a context in which all have benefited, have produced a highly
differentiated set of economic consequences in which the claims of privatisation,
even on its own terms, have not always been achieved [document 13]. At the
same time, and most significantly for the policy areas which form the core of
this book, economic privatisation has been accompanied by a set of developments which have allowed the obligations placed upon powerful companies to
be circumvented and the consequences privatised into the lives of those who
can bear those consequences the least.

PART TWO

Chapter 4

HOUSING

The second part of this book opens with a chapter which deals with the impact of privatisation upon housing policy and provision. While it is arguably the aspect of welfare in which the state has played the smallest role, privatisation can claim both to have originated in the housing field and to have had a more substantial impact here than in any other area.

While the direct involvement of the state in housing provision was of a different order from its intervention in education, health or social security, the connection between privatisation and housing was a more powerful one. The Conservative Party Manifesto at the 1979 General Election contained one and a half pages outlining a housing policy which concentrated almost exclusively upon issues of ownership and the sale of council houses. As such, it received more attention than any other social policy area. Forrest (1993: 40) suggests that 'the Right to Buy was one of the few fully worked out privatisation policies in the 1979 Conservative Manifesto'. The particular version of privatisation represented by the policy needs careful attention. The sale of council housing did not emanate from the New Right preoccupations with liberalisation and marketisation, but was part of the long-standing Conservative ideological preference for private over public ownership and in its more recent determination to cut-back public expenditure and to narrow the scope of the local state. The early policy of new administration towards housing was thus firmly located in the more general drive towards the privatisation of property. In the latter half of the 1980s, as this chapter will show, the emphasis was to switch away from property itself and towards the privatisation of choice and the development of market relations.

The combined impact of privatisation approaches in this area of policy was to be profound. In terms of its impact upon individuals, for example, Plumridge (1996: 129) suggests that 'lifestyles are much more likely to be altered by the privatisation of housing than by the combined effects of all other privatisations'. At a broader policy level, Forrest and Murie (1993: i), among many other commentators, suggest that, 'In social, political and economic terms, the most important element in the privatisation programme of the Thatcher governments has been the sale of publicly-owned housing.' This importance derives both from timing – housing privatisation was in the vanguard of a far wider policy development – and scope. The sale of council housing, as this chapter will later demonstrate, generated receipts on a scale unrivalled by any other transfer of assets from public to private hands.

4.1 What did the Conservatives inherit?

Chapter 2 of this book suggested that the drive towards privatisation in the 1980s was based, at least in part, upon the criticisms of public services which had grown up over more than a decade. These criticisms were to be found at both the right and left of the political spectrum and were certainly present in the field of housing. Smith *et al.* (1996: 290), for example, suggest 'the provision of large-scale non-traditional public housing in the 1960s is widely regarded as an expensive and unpopular failure, which has had detrimental effects on the lives of council tenants . . . and the management of public housing has often left a great deal to be desired, certainly from the tenant's perspective.' On parts of the Left, too, council housing was portrayed as inefficient and repressive, a tool of social policing rather than empowerment. Even when physical conditions were of a good standard, as was generally the case, the treatment of tenants, in terms of choice and influence, was of a far lesser order. The positive case for the sale of council houses could plausibly be portrayed as part of a wider effort to free tenants from the political stranglehold of insensitive, self-interested housing authorities.

As Smith *et al.* (1996: 287) suggest, the approach developed by the 1979 administration fell within 'a programme of replacing welfare state systems of collective provision and public funding with more individual and privatised systems [and] . . . an ideological opposition to the direct public provision of services'. For the first time, social housing, and council housing in particular, appeared in public policy as a housing problem to be solved, rather than as a solution to housing problems. In its more extreme formulations, council housing appeared in the speeches of government Ministers as not only a problem in its own right, but as a cause of difficulties in other social spheres. Forrest and Murie (1993: 12) quote Housing Minister Geoffrey Pattie, in 1986, as asserting that 'Council housing breeds slums, delinquency, vandalism, waste, arrears and social polarisation'.

The 1980 Housing Act, with which Conservative policy began, replaced concern over housing supply and quality by a focus upon tenure and the clearing of any local impediments which might have been placed in the path of those wishing to exercise the new Right To Buy (RTB). A new uniform statutory procedure, replacing former local voluntary discretion, was backed up by extensive powers of intervention by the Secretary of State, in order to ensure compliance. Tenants of at least three years' standing were to be provided with a statutory eligibility to buy at market discounts of a minimum of 33 per cent, with an additional percentage point for each year of tenancy beyond three years, up to a maximum of 50 per cent. The Act backed up these rights with the guarantee of a mortgage for potential purchasers. It led to a level of sales which

Table 4.1 Sales of dwellings by local authorities: 1979–1982, England and Wales

Year	All sales of dwellings
1979	41,665
1980	81,485
1981	102,825
1982	201,880

Source: *Housing and Construction Statistics*, HMSO

surpassed anything achieved under former arrangements and continued to expand over the next two years.

When sales began to slow in 1983, a series of further Acts, in the successive years of 1984, 1985 and 1986, introduced new measures to stimulate sales. The Housing and Building Control Act reduced the residential qualification from three years to two, bringing some 250,000 additional tenants within the right to buy. For tenants of thirty years standing, the maximum discount was increased from 50 to 60 per cent. For tenants of flats – which had proved relatively unattractive to potential purchasers – discounts now began at 44 per cent and increased to 70 per cent after only 15 years' tenancy. Early resale penalties were reduced, children succeeding to their parents' tenancies were provided with a statutory, rather than discretionary, right to discounts and the procedures which landlords had to follow under the right to buy were tightened up, to allow less room for delay. Other measures, outside the RTB framework itself, added to the pressures towards purchase. Mortgage Interest Tax Relief, for example, increased the attractiveness of home buying at the same time as the Government pursued a policy of raising rents sharply in the public sector.

For those unable to purchase, a switch in government expenditure from bricks and mortar to Housing Benefit formed part of an attempt to operate a market in the rented sector. As Lund (1996: 179) noted, it provided 'a form of income-related voucher for rented accommodation that is transferable between homes'. As the same author suggests, however, the theory and practice were only imperfectly matched in this regard:

'A social security system based only on income [and not therefore sensitive to different rent levels in different places] would cause considerable hardship to those living in high rent areas but the logic of a free market dictates that people with low incomes should not be living in such areas.'

4.2 Results of the Right to Buy

Results of RTB for pubic authorities

The privatisation policy produced a series of consequences for public authorities. At local council level, the main effect was in the loss of stock previously available for rent. By 1995, as Balchin *et al.* (1998: 68) show, a total of 1,569,321 council dwellings had been sold over the previous fifteen years, equivalent to 25 per cent of the total housing stock of 1980. Nor were these dwellings drawn uniformly from the whole of the council housing. Sales were concentrated among the more desirable properties, both in terms of physical condition and location. Councils were not only left with diminishing numbers of dwellings but the overall quality of stock was also poorer than before the Right to Buy policy had begun.

The positive impact of sales was to be found in the generation of capital receipts. The sums raised through sales were substantial and, particularly in early phases, outstripped any other element in the government's privatisation programme. Forrest and Murie (1993: 93) show that housing capital receipts between 1979/80 and 1985/86 totalled £9,527 million while other privatisation activities, taken all together, generated £7,732 million. The same authors conclude (1993: 254–5) that,

'In the ten years 1979–89 capital receipts from the housing programme were some £17.5 billion. This compared with £23.5 billion from all the privatisation policies. Housing receipts represented 43% of all privatisation proceeds and was both the largest and most sustained source of capital receipts.'

The massive scale of the receipts involved in house privatisation should not, however, draw attention away from the scale of inducements which were paid from the public purse to purchasers. The gap between the market value of council properties and the price charged under the RTB grew steadily as the need to attract more purchasers became more acute. The value of discounts in 1986, for example, amounted to £5.6 billion. By 1990 , when the average discount had risen to 53 per cent, a further £2.5 billion was added to the financial cost of the sales policy (Kemp 1992).

Results of RTB for individuals

If the Right to Buy thus involved financial costs, as well as gains, for public authorities, the same pattern can be found in relation to individuals. Balchin *et al.* (1998: 68) translate the global costs of discounts into individual terms in this way: 'It was clear that local authority tenants who had exercised the RTB had been the recipients of the largest housing subsidy of all, averaging £12,094 nationally, and as much as £21,675 in London.' The contrast between the essentially Schumpeterian nature of council house sales – with its emphasis upon the benefits of private ownership *per se* – and the marketising preoccupations of the neo-liberals emerge clearly in this way. Lund (1996: 49) suggests that the whole process 'seems distant from the philosophy of free markets advocated by Hayek – a true marketeer would have sold the houses on vacant possession at full market value'. Forrest and Murie (1993: 267) assess the ideological basis of the policy as 'less as a triumph of privatisation and more as a massive shift in the nature and pattern of state subsidy in housing – from the poorest to the better off'.

Kemp (1992: 65) quotes the 1987 Conservative Party Manifesto as describing home ownership as 'the great success story of housing policy' *[document 4]*. Yet, the slow-down in sales themselves, and a growing questioning of the free-market credentials of the Right to Buy policy, were bringing about serious changes in the government's approach. While the privatisation approach had, undoubtedly, asserted the preference for individualism over collectivism and produced a shift in favour of housing being provided as part of the private market, it had yet to make substantial inroads into the creation of choice and diversity for those who were likely to remain as public tenants. Whereas the RTB policy had its roots outside the influential New Right, the application of ideas from that quarter to housing policy had not been neglected. Smith *et al.* (1996: 290) quote Pennance and Gray (1968), for example, as arguing that:

'If there are no restrictions on price, consumer choice or the entry of new producers or sellers, a strongly competitive market will ensure that the size, quantity and quality of houses that are built and the distribution of existing stock will be dictated by the tastes, incomes and preferences of consumers.'

As the thrust towards marketisation gathered pace during the middle years of the 1980s, these arguments emerged once again in relation to housing. Thus a 1985 publication of the Adam Smith Institute argued that

'There is scope . . . for taking the whole problem of housing out of the local political arena, and contriving a situation in which both ownership and rent are regulated not by political whim but by demand for it and the supply which can be generated to meet it.' (Butler *et al.* 1985: 43)

4.3 Reforms in the second half of the 1980s onwards

The effect of the changing climate was evident in the Housing and Planning Act 1986 which, while further extending discounts to sitting tenants and again streamlining the application procedure, also allowed for the sale of whole estates or property portfolios to be made to private housing trusts and to new landlords. The shift of emphasis was away from individual preferences in relation to tenure and towards a more emphatic de-municipalisation. The Conservative Party Manifesto of 1987 carried the suggestion further in its declaration that, 'We will give each council house tenant individually the right to transfer the ownership of his or her house to a housing association or other independent, approved landlord.' The determination to create a variety of different arrangements for ownership and control within the housing market had come to occupy the centre ground of government policy making. Butcher (1995: 101) quotes the then-Minister for Housing, William Waldegrave (1987: 8), as suggesting that, 'the next great push after the right to buy should be to get rid of the State as a big landlord and bring housing back to the community'.

In this new climate, a series of liberalising policy initiatives were now applied to housing. Smith *et al.* (1996: 307) summarise the changes in this period as follows: 'The emphasis has been placed upon financial controls, increasing competitions, market mechanisms, privatisation, a contract culture, service quality and performance management, with the citizen viewed as the consumer.' In terms of the preoccupations of this book, these themes will be familiar as part of the core curriculum of the New Right free marketeers. The problematisation of the local and the political, and the promotion of market mechanisms as uncomplicated solutions, fitted well with existing government dislike of council housing, while allowing that hostility to be carried further. Not only was property to be privatised, but the processes of production, provision and management could be placed in private hands as well.

The outcome of the 1987 General Election led to a fresh impetus in translating these ideas into practical action in the housing field. Lund (1996: 51) suggests that a major reappraisal of policy and strategy was evident in a post-election White Paper and in its four aims for the future, which he summarises as: 'First to reverse the decline of private rented housing and improve its quality: second to give council tenants the right to transfer to other landlords if they choose to do so; third to target money more accurately on the most acute problems; and fourth to continue to promote the growth of owner occupation' (DoE 1987: 3). The Housing Act 1988 and the Local Government and Housing Act 1989 quickly followed. A further reshaping of the public/private boundary followed when new tax incentives were introduced for private landlords. This direct use of public money to promote private provision illustrates some of the complexity of the relationship between the two sectors. Privatisation was not identical with reductions in public expenditure. As Kemp (1992: 71) suggests, 'Previous attempts to revive the private landlord were based very largely on deregulating rents. Thus while the objective was not new, subsidizing the private landlord was a distinctively different policy instrument of Mrs Thatcher's Governments.'

As discussed more fully in Chapter 6, the marketeers' preference for 'exit' over 'voice' in exercising influence over services resulted in tenants being given the right, known as 'Tenants' Choice', to ballot in order to leave local authority control and choose a different landlord. The strength of feeling among ministers that tenants were trapped within a welfare system produced a voting system which was widely regarded as containing an in-built bias against council control. In any ballot concerning a possible transfer, those eligible to vote, but not doing so, were taken to be in favour of the new landlord, rather than the local authority.

In addition to Tenants' Choice, the 1988 reforms contained one further new initiative by which ministers placed great store. The Housing Action Trust (HAT) programme was to provide a means of directing central government funds for repair and renovation, without the involvement of local authorities. It was, Lund (1996: 51) suggests, 'a vital part of the government's housing policy'. In July 1988, the government announced its intention of setting up a three-year programme, funded with £125 million. Lambeth, Southwark, Tower Hamlets,

Leeds, Sandwell and Southwark were identified as areas where HATs might first be established. The original proposal included no mechanism for balloting tenants on the HAT proposals. When that right was conceded, it marked the effective end of the policy as, in practice, the idea was consistently rejected by tenants who, despite the large sums of money on offer, did not wish, as Forrest (1993: 43) suggests, 'to exit from the council sector regardless of the destination'. The uncertainty of housing association management – particularly in relation to rent levels – or the prospect of returning to private landlords, from whom many council tenants had spent long years attempting to escape, combined to make the virtues of diversity less attractive than the free marketeers had supposed. The smack of privatisation and the conjured up images of private landlordism were, according to Smith *et al.* (1996: 298), sufficient to produce such a direct contradiction of the calculation of individual advantage which the privatisers had presupposed. Tenants' Choice met the same fate, being abandoned as a scheme in 1995.

Kemp (1992: 74), in considering the fate of HATs and Tenants' Choice, concludes that failure lay in the concept rather than the execution:

'The Government assumed that disgruntled council tenants would rush at the opportunity to change their landlord. But while council tenants are keen enough to enter the market at a reduced price when the commodity on offer is the ownership of their own home, they do not do so when it comes to renting it. The advantages to them in renting from a private sector landlord appeared limited but the disadvantages – much reduced security of tenure, a more punitive attitude to arrears and the prospect of higher rents – seemed significant.'

Supporters of the initiatives were left to point to the not-inconsiderable benefit which had resulted in changing the balance of power between tenants and local authority landlords. The availability of choice, it was said, had produced an incentive among existing providers to improve their performance. The argument remained at a considerable remove, however, from the promises of large-scale, tenant-initiated change with which the programmes had been launched.

The absence of a popular mandate led, among those councils for whom privatisation was an attractive proposition, to an alternative means of achieving some of the sought-after elimination of local authorities from the provider role. Large Scale Voluntary Transfer (LSVT), as it came to be known, emerged during the 1990s. It involved a local authorities-initiated transfer of the whole of their housing stock to new housing associations, some of which they themselves had set up. Such plans generally emanated from council officers and politicians, rather than tenants themselves, for whom the transfer usually involved the exchange of one monopoly landlord for another. For councils, the advantages lay in the generation of capital receipts and, until the Housing Act 1996 when the position was reversed, the fact that tenants of the new housing associations were not eligible for the Right To Buy. As a result of the policy, Walker (1997: 76) estimates that 52 local authorities had transferred the whole of their stock in this way, moving nearly a quarter of a million homes into the housing association sector.

One of the essential switches in housing policy during the second half of the 1980s was to be found in the increasing prominence accorded to housing associations, as opposed to local authorities, in the provision of social housing. These organisations had already undergone a significant change in character in the 1974 Housing Act which had transformed their previous voluntary character to one where the volume of state support and subsidy located them firmly within the public sector, albeit with continuing strong voluntary roots. Using the public subsidy, Plumridge (1996: 134) argues that the Conservative administrations of the 1980s changed the character of housing associations again, as part of the 'privatisation of housing production', to a position where they became 'dominant in the production of social housing'.

This development was given a further twist in the 1988 Housing Act which introduced a new private finance regime for housing associations. As a result, associations were obliged to raise over one-third of the funding required for building projects from private financial markets. Exposure to the 'disciplines of the market' (DoE 1987) would emphasise again the nature of the agencies as closer to private than public forms of organisation and operation, entrenching a new agenda of markets, competition, entrepreneurship and private management techniques.

Housing remained a field in which legislative activity continued throughout the Conservative administration of 1992–97. As the supply of tenants exercising the Right to Buy slowed further, by 1996 reaching the lowest recorded level since the inception of the policy in 1980 (Wilcox 1997b: 43), the 1992 Conservative Manifesto promised a new scheme of converting Rents to Mortgage which, as Smith et al. (1996: 302) suggest, 'allowed tenants to convert their rental payment into a mortgage payment and to receive a discount on the value of the property'. The scheme was directed at the 1.25 million council tenants not in receipt of housing benefit although, as Lund (1996: 182) reports, by 1995 only 11 of them had chosen to do so.

Within the public rented sector, the introduction of 'market testing' into local authority housing management proceeded according to the mechanisms of competitive tendering. The result, it has been suggested, has been for housing management in many local authorities to become 'reformed from within' (Cole and Furbey 1994: 217). Butcher (1995: 110) identifies the key features of such reforms as being the decentralisation of the housing service and the development of more customer-oriented approaches. Such reforms, however, took place within a context where public investment in housing continued to bear the largest burden of cuts in capital programmes – an approach which had been characteristic of the Conservative approach from 1979 onwards. Now, as Wilcox (1997b: 51) suggests, housing was again 'put at the end of the queue compared to other services, as overall public spending was squeezed to make way for a reduction in income tax rates. Provision for housing investment has been reduced progressively for some years; the cut-backs announced in the 1996 Budget were, however, far more severe than in previous years.' In privatisation terms, as the same author observes, the cuts were justified by the increased reliance which the government placed upon its Private Finance Initiative to shift capital borrowing for infrastructure investments into the private sector, and outside the PSBR.

For Housing Associations, too, change continued throughout the first half of the 1990s. The 1996 Housing Act abandoned the name itself in favour of the Registered Social Landlord sector. In part, at least, this change recognised the impact of the large-scale voluntary transfer of local authority housing departments into the association sector, as discussed above. By the time of the Act, according to Walker (1997: 76), a quarter of all homes in the registered social landlord sector were ex-local authority homes. In a consultation paper issued in February 1997, it was suggested by government that all housing authorities should, in future, have to include stock transfer proposals in their housing strategies (Malpass 1998: 179).

By 1997, therefore, policy in the housing field had pursued a privatisation and marketisation agenda to the point where a series of very important changes had been achieved. The pattern of housing tenure had shifted decisively in favour of home ownership, rather than renting. Owner-occupation rose, as a share of total housing stock, from 52 per cent in 1979 to 67 per cent in 1995. Within the rented sector, the nature of local authority provision was much altered. In common with its approach in other social policy areas, the Conservative intention had been to transform councils into strategic arm's-length enablers and regulators, rather than providers, of services. Tenants were to be consumers, rather than clients, exercising choice in a market diversified by a revived private rented sector, the promotion of housing associations and the pervasive introduction of private sector management techniques which Walker (1997: 74) summarises as, 'output-based accounting, rather than input-based; incentives and contracts for performance rather than trust-based relationships; quasi-markets and disaggregated units replacing planning and provision structures; the introduction of competition from all sectors; and the promotion of exit over voice as user influence'.

4.4 Making an assessment

This chapter now turns to an assessment of the strategies and practical approaches outlined above. There can be no doubt that, especially during the first half of the period between 1979 and 1997, the thrust away from the public and towards the private provision of housing represented a major enterprise for the Conservative governments and one through which the landscape of housing in Britain was profoundly affected. While, as Burchardt (1997) confirms, the private provision of housing was of a different order from that in education or health throughout the period, the element which could be considered 'purely private' accounted for 58 per cent of the housing sector in 1979/80 and rose by more than 10 per cent to 69 per cent in 1995/96. The 'pure public' sector was correspondingly small: 18 per cent in 1979/80, falling to 10 per cent by 1995/56.

In the latter half of the Conservative period, however, when the New Right came more into an ascendancy, the approach to housing policy faltered. In some areas, initiatives failed in their own terms. Both Tenants' Choice and Housing Action Trusts foundered when individual tenants failed to become the active market seekers that those framing these policies had predicted. Rent-to-Mortgage proved to be far less attractive without the direct financial incentive which had accompanied the earlier Right to Buy schemes. More significantly, the policy of reviving the private rented sector, which had formed a consistent threat in government policy, also failed to produce its intended results. The basic belief that the market, once set free from regulation, would revive of its own accord, proved to be an over-simplification. As Kemp (1992: 75) suggests, deregulation was at most a necessary and certainly not a sufficient condition for revival. In any case, the market for private renting could not be sealed from the effects of government policy in other parts of the housing field. The taxation and other financial privileges used to promote the policy of home ownership made renting, whether public or private, appear a second-best form of tenure.

As well as policies which fail within their own terms, however, the effects of policies which themselves succeed have to be considered in relation to other policy areas. Three need to receive attention here:

- What happened to people who bought their own homes?
- What happened to people who remained in the public rented sector?
- What happened to people who had no homes at all?

People who bought their own homes

As suggested earlier in this chapter, individuals who exercised the Right to Buy, at least in the initial phases, found themselves in receipt of a substantial subsidy and in possession of an appreciating asset. By the end of the Conservative era, however, the nature of home ownership had altered significantly, and the notion that 'property owning' was somehow a higher form of tenure, conferring social status, had come under considerable question. The impact of privatisation upon the credit industry – through deregulation – had brought home ownership within the reach of a far wider spectrum of income. As far as individuals are concerned, Wilcox and Ford (1997: 24–5) assess the situation in the second half of the 1990s in this way:

> 'with some two-thirds of all households now home-owners, by definition it is far from being the exclusive preserve of only the most affluent households in society . . . home-buyers now make up two-fifths of all households in the lower half of the bottom income decile. In 1979 they made up just 14% of the households in that lowest income band. . . . More generally, one in six home-buying households do not have household heads in full-time employment, twice as many as there were at the beginning of the 1980s.'

The onset of globalisation during the 1980s and the recession of the first part of the 1990s meant, moreover, that even for households with employment, the nature of work had become more unreliable and the prospects of sustaining employment over the lifetime of a mortgage harder to gauge. Wilcox and Ford (1997: 25) point out that current best estimates suggest that, over the course of a year, more than half a million home-buying households will experience a period of unemployment by at least one mortgagor. Moreover, the period of time between losing one job and obtaining another is lengthening, and the proportion of those who fail to find work again within a twelve-month period is growing.

The economic recession of the early 1990s produced a severe impact upon the housing market. High mortgage arrears and repossessions grew at a rate which Malpass (1998: 182) records as, 'never before experienced in Britain'. Figures provided by Ford (1997: 88) show that, in 1981, 4,870 households lost their homes in this manner. By 1987, the figure was 26,390 and in 1991 the numbers peaked at 75,540. Even following the recovery of the middle of the decade the situation has failed to return to pre-recession levels. At the same time, negative equity and low inflation rates – which failed to produce the rapidly reducing repayment-to-earnings ratios of earlier periods – meant that struggling households were less able to take advantage of 'trading down' within the housing market or exiting from it altogether.

It was against this background that the administration of 1992 implemented a further strand in the government's portfolio of privatisation measures. The strategy was one of shifting the responsibility for meeting particular costs from the state to the individual. For private house purchasers, the social security system had, under certain conditions, provided for assistance with mortgage interest payments at times of unemployment. As the costs associated with this scheme rose during the recession, the Minister responsible for Social Security, Peter Lilley, moved to lessen the assistance available from the state, and to promote an alternative of personal provision, organised through the private insurance market. These changes were part of a wider policy thrust in social security and health policy in favour of private insurance-based provision, as Chapters 5 and 9 demonstrate.

The main changes in the nature and level of state support took place in October 1995. Ford and Kempson (1997) for the Joseph Rowntree Foundation reviewed the practical impact which followed. The authors conclude that the market had failed to respond in the way which New Right thinkers might have envisaged: 'Few new private insurance products have been developed to mirror the cuts to State provision . . . there have been few innovative products.' Consumers, too, had proved less than enthusiastic about covering their own risks. Take-up of insurance to cover periods of unemployment rose by some 3–4 percentage points between 1994 and 1996, adding some 5 or 6 per cent to average mortgage costs. Markets, as Chapter 3 suggested, operate in ways which have potential deficits in terms of equity and universal coverage. In this instance, as Ford and Kempson discovered, 'the research indicates a poor alignment between risk and taking insurance. . . . Grossing up the figures, this indicates a potential 2.5 million borrowers without insurance.' Nor do insurance policies in relation to potential unemployment provide a solution to the majority of income support claimants in receipt of help with mortgage costs at the time when eligibility for help was reduced. Individuals requiring assistance because of disability, retirement or lone parenthood made up two-thirds of those in receipt of help with mortgage interest payments in May 1995. Insurance provision for unemployment is of no relevance to individuals in these circumstances, while the changes in benefit entitlement affect all claimants.

The impact of market forces, and the privatisation of their consequences, brought about a sea-change in public attitudes towards private home ownership by the end of the Conservative period in office. The 14th British Social Attitudes Report (Jowell, 1997) asked respondents about the potential disadvantages of home ownership. Over a decade, the percentage who believed that home ownership now involved a substantial element of risk had doubled from 25 to 50 per cent. One of the pivotal claims of privatisation, that private ownership would of itself produce new levels of individual satisfaction while stimulating the qualities of active citizenship, was thus called into question.

Those who remained in the rented sector

For those who remained in the rented sector the impact of privatisation in housing policy was sharper still. The continuing efforts to increase the flow of private rented accommodation – through liberalisation, tax concessions and so on – had proved unsuccessful. Williams (1992: 168) estimates that 50,000 to 60,000 units for private rental were lost each year during the 1980s. The most striking effect, in the public sphere, was in terms of social polarisation. Figures from the London School of Economics (1998) suggest that, by 1994, 76 per cent of those in council housing were in the poorest two-fifths of the population, compared to 51 per cent in 1979. Market forces have produced a pattern of social and spatial polarisation, in which, as Forrest and Murie (1993: 174) suggest, 'British council housing is becoming the form of housing provision for those excluded from the mainstream of social consumption'. The effect of policy changes during the 1980s and early 1990s was thus to exaggerate the partial nature of public housing and to emphasise the contrast which always existed between the housing field and the provision of more universal social policy services, such as education and health.

Nor are these features confined to local authority provision. The introduction of private financing into housing association funding necessitated, in real terms, rises in the rents charged to association tenants. The provision of means-tested housing benefit to meet these increased charges had the effect of creating an unemployment trap, effectively eliminating any worthwhile financial gain which might have been forthcoming through taking up employment. Wilcox (1997a) shows that the proportion of employed tenants entering the housing association sector declined rapidly from 52 per cent in 1984 to just 27 per cent in 1995/96.

Social and spatial polarisation, as Lund (1996: 185) suggests, is an inevitable component of market operation: 'Markets allocate dwellings according to ability to pay and, because location is by far the most important determinant of house prices, then markets generate spatial polarisation.' The spatial consequences of privatisation occur across the boundaries of particular services. They are, as Chapter 3 suggested, a particular feature of the privatisation of the utilities. Bartlett *et al.* (1998: 4), in their overview of quasi-market reforms, similarly conclude that,

> 'With the devolution of decision-making and of responsibility of individual provider units, the quality and style of provision varies by location. In many sectors of welfare services it is apparent that the quality of services depends as much on where users live as on the level of need which they experience, creating both winners and losers from the reforms.'

Thus, the impact of polarisation extends far beyond the housing sphere. Housing outcomes meet and combine with the spatial consequences of privatisation in other policy areas. As Lund (1996: 185) puts it, housing consequences have 'significant implications for equality of educational opportunity, racial equality, law and order and social integration'. The particular point to emphasise here is that Bartlett *et al.*'s 'winners and losers' do not emerge haphazardly in these circumstances. Rather, losses are concentrated in particular places, and among particular groups, while the gains are siphoned off to the already-advantaged.

Social and economic detriment of public renting took place, ironically, at a time when – in considering the shifting boundary of public and private provision – the sector became a net contributor to the public purse rather than a demand upon it. In 1979 a letter sent by one of Mrs Thatcher's aides to a constituent who had complained about the state of repair of her council house suggested that 'considering the fact you have been unable to buy your own accommodation you are lucky to have been given something which the rest of us are paying for out of our taxes' (quoted in *The Times*, 9 April 1979). By 1994/ 95, this position was quite reversed. Rather than the private circumstances of local authority renters being subsidised by the public, council housing as a whole in Great Britain has generated a net surplus which, in 1996, totalled over £550 million, and was projected to grow still further (Wilcox 1997b: 61).

A considerable proportion of the surplus noted above, however, was derived from another part of the public purse – the housing benefit system. The rise in housing benefit expenditure had been a planned part of the government's decision to switch policy away from subsidising the building of new housing. The impact of that switch, however, had been greater than anticipated, especially outside the council sector. As Malpass (1998: 180) explains:

> 'Rent allowances (covering private and housing association tenants) grew at an annual rate of 22 per cent between 1988/9 and 1993/4; this compared with only 7.6 per cent for local authority rent rebate expenditure. Private sector tenants constituted just over a third of all housing benefit claimants but their rent levels meant that they accounted for nearly half of all housing benefit expenditure.'

In an attempt to place some constraint upon the escalation of expenditure in the private market, the government introduced new housing benefit rules in January 1996. A cap was to be placed on rents deemed to be in excess of the average for the locality. Additional restrictions applied to single people aged under 25. The changes were intended to work, according to the market theorists by whom they were introduced, by strengthening the hand of tenants to negotiate rents downwards or, failing that, by obliging them to find cheaper accommodation. In a market where demand exceeded supply, however, these were always unlikely outcomes. A report from the housing charity Shelter (1998) provided evidence that private landlords were refusing to rent to young people because of the benefit cuts. The changes brought about were thus upon the behaviour of the provider, not the purchaser. The provision of private rented accommodation slowed in the period after the changes were introduced, thus undermining one of the most consistently stated housing policy goals of all Conservative administrations.

If the effect of privatisation and marketisation upon those left in the rented sector has been to marginalise and residualise, the impact has been greater still upon those who have been unable to gain a foothold within any form of housing tenure. Forrest (1993: 50) suggests that, in the housing field, the injection of the vocabulary and practices of the market has been targeted at a group whose previous experience has been as 'casualties of market processes and generally have weak market positions as both producers and consumers'. The most vulnerable of these groups are those without homes at all, as the remainder of this chapter now demonstrates.

Those who have no homes at all

For official policy makers during the first decade of Thatcher administrations homelessness was an issue which barely figured upon the housing agenda. While figures for homelessness grew, the 1987 Housing White Paper failed to mention the problem at all. The scale of the issue is outlined by Kemp (1992: 77) who suggests that 'during the 1980s the number of homeless people increased considerably, creating a "third nation" in housing . . . the number of households accepted for rehousing because of homelessness increased from 53,110 in 1978 to 126,680 in 1989 or 139%'. The scale of homelessness continued to increase during the 1990s. Wilcox (1996) records that the number of homeless households in Great Britain accepted by local authorities rose from about 70,000 in 1979 to 179,000 in 1992.

The sale of local authority accommodation and the effective elimination of council building of new homes for rent combined to make the response to growing homelessness even more problematic. With a decline in the stock of social rented housing in Britain of more than a quarter between 1979 and 1995 (Malpass 1998: 177), the use of bed and breakfast or other forms of temporary accommodation increased sharply from less than 3,000 at the start of the 1980s to nearly 38,000 at its close (Kemp 1992: 77). In this way, while public expenditure on providing decent and affordable accommodation had been reduced, it has been replaced by profit making in the private bed and breakfast sector. As Forrest and Murie (1993: 265) put it, this outcome 'is a prime example of ideology overriding hard economic considerations'.

Nor does the impact of privatisation upon homelessness end there. Shelter Cymru (1996: 1), for example, in an analysis of Welsh Office statistics, estimate that for every household accepted as homeless by Welsh local authorities, another two fail entirely to obtain help from the system. The social policy shifts of the post-1979 period worked in a way which did not simply transfer property and functions from the public to private hands. It also, as Chapter 3 demonstrated in relation to the utilities, privatised the consequences of policy decisions, by removing responsibilities which had hitherto been accepted within the public sphere, leaving households and individuals to deal with the results as best they could. These are deliberate policy actions and are as apparent in housing as in any other social policy field Pressure upon local authorities, for example, led during the 1980s and 1990s to a tightening of the criteria by which families might be accepted as homeless and a diminution in the services which might then be offered to them. As Stewart (1998: 53) suggests, the outcome is one of exclusion, brought about by 'discriminatory policies and procedures which set priorities and deny access to certain groups, or offer them only the worst housing available'. Figures published by the government, which cover the last quarter before the implementation of the changes brought about by the 1996 Housing Act, show that the acceptances of people presenting themselves as homeless had dropped dramatically in most parts of Wales and England. Compared to a year earlier, for example, there had been a 26 per cent fall in acceptances in Wales and the North East of England. Thus, even before the newly restricted rights came into being, the practical help available to the most vulnerable had been contracting rapidly.

In the 1996 Housing Act, the government repealed the rights of homeless people to priority rehousing, on the basis that it gave them an unfair advantage over those on council waiting lists. Instead, the responsibility of local authorities to those found unintentionally homeless was to provide only temporary accommodation for a two-year period (Harriott and Matthews 1998: 156). At the same time, the new Act provided social landlords with more control over the allocation of tenancies, with a broad level of discretion to determine 'what classes of person are, or are not' to be regarded as qualified for housing. For those who were successful in being offered a home, the use of 'introductory' tenancies, offered a less secure form of tenure than in the past. Thereafter, councils were provided with new and greater powers to evict those already in occupation.

The powers of the 1996 Act came into force on 1 April 1997, representing one of the final acts in the eighteen-year history of Conservative government. Butler (1998), in a report for the housing charity Shelter, published an account of her investigations of the practical implementation of the new powers during their first year. It found that the policy of privatising social problems had escalated rapidly during the twelve-month period. While over half the local author-ities surveyed were unable to provide figures of those excluded or suspended from their housing registers, the 44 authorities able to do so had excluded a total of 32,971 households, suggesting a national figure of some 200,000. The total of recorded exclusions and suspensions was four times greater in 1997/98 than in the previous year. While the legislation under which such actions were undertaken had been framed largely in an atmosphere of rising public concern and media concentration upon 'neighbours from hell', sex offenders and crime on estates (Goodwin 1998), exclusions for antisocial behaviour were actually a small minority, at just 3 per cent of households. Rather, refusal to house was dominated by rent arrears (accounting for 36 per cent of excluded households), owner-occupation and insufficient length of residence in the local authority area. Ford (1997: 91) explores these outcomes in relation to owner-occupation, in particular – the form of tenure most actively promoted during the Conservat-ive era. Her conclusion is that 'housing policy, together with fiscal and wider economic measures, came together first to facilitate the expansion of house-holds' access to home ownership and then to jeopardize households' ability to maintain their financial commitments'. Only 30 per cent of households under-going repossession, and no more than 50 per cent of those where repossession followed a court order, were accepted for rehousing by the local authority while, as Ford (1997: 89) put it, 'the percentage of those in possession, and rehoused following acceptance as officially homeless, has been falling'.

Commenting on the Shelter report, Goodwin (1998: 26), concluded that the effect of the 1996 Act, 'is that people are being excluded from ever getting an opportunity of social housing'. The basis of this exclusion was often an undifferentiated policy which denied the consideration of individual circum-stances. Moreover, the level of verification required by councils was, in just under half of those responding, one of 'belief', rather than 'proof'. The combina-tion of restrictive tenancy powers, and the diminution of rights of homeless people, often resulted in such applications being dealt with as general housing applications, rather than under the homelessness legislation. In the conclusion of Shelter's director, the result has been the exclusion not of people 'who are dangerous, or guilty of antisocial behaviour – we are looking at wide-ranging and sometimes indiscriminate policies.' The consequences of these policies lie where they fall – privatised into the lives of those least able to bear the consequences.

4.5 Summary

Malpass (1998: 184) suggests that, 'in housing perhaps more than any other part of the welfare state', the Conservative years were characterised by sticking to the mantra of 'private good, public bad'. Quite certainly, the unifying thread in all the changes outlined in this chapter has been the shift in responsibility for housing provision from the public to the private spheres. This change often involved the direct transfer of large sums of public money in order to advance this end, even at a time when, as Lowe (1993) demonstrates, housing suffered the greatest cut-backs of all the major social services, during the Conservative years since 1979. To a greater extent, perhaps, than in any other social policy area, the 'strategic jigsaw' (Sullivan 1996: 45) in housing policy had, through a combination of its different elements, produced an outcome in which the future appeared only fit for further gains along the road to private provision. By 1998, the process had gone so far that Glennerster and Hills (1998) suggest that housing policy *per se* had virtually disappeared as a distinct area for study, being 'mainly now an adjunct of social security and city regeneration strategies'. In that process, as this chapter has demonstrated, the advantages and disadvantages of policies pursued have fallen unevenly and, in some ways, unpredictably upon those affected. The substitution of market forces for planned intervention by government has produced benefits for those best able to exploit them, while heaping disadvantageous consequences upon those who have least resources from which they might be borne. From a basis where, as suggested at the start of this chapter, the provision of a decent home for every family had generally been regarded as part of the basic responsibility of the state, the ideological stance of government had become one where that responsibility had been transferred to the market for those who could prosper within it, and where those who could not were left to their own salvation.

Chapter 5

SOCIAL SECURITY

The application of privatisation and marketisation approaches may appear, at first inspection, to have played a lesser part in the post-1979 history of social security policy than in the other major social dimensions considered in this book. Bradshaw (1992: 99), for example, suggests that, from a Right Wing perspective, the Thatcher governments 'never really got round to social security'. The argument presented in this chapter, by contrast, will suggest that while income maintenance might have proved more intractable to reform, this did not prevent it from being the focus of sustained and consistent attention by policy makers. It occupies second place in the sequence of chapters in this part because of the full role played within it, by what Dean (1993: 86), in his discussion of social security policy, describes as the 'shifting balance between the state (i.e. collective) and individual (i.e. private) provision'. By the end of the eighteen years of Conservative administration, members of the neo-liberal wing of its politics could, with justice, claim that while individual changes might appear 'relatively minor', the final result had been 'radical change' (Pirie 1995).

5.1 Early reforms

While the full range of reforms in this field were only to become apparent as time unfolded, the essential thread in government policies was to remain consistent throughout. One of the earliest changes involved the privatisation of sickness benefit, in which it was proposed, in 1980, to replace national insurance sickness benefit for employees during short-term sickness absence, with statutory sick pay, administered by employers. The Departmental White Paper (DHSS 1980: 2) which proposed the change suggested that government should 'disengage itself from activities which firms and individuals can perform perfectly well for themselves'. Fifteen years later, in recognisably the same language, the then-Secretary of State for Social Security set out the basis of his own approach as rooted in the belief that 'private welfare strengthens the economy while taxpayer financed welfare weakens it' (Lilley 1995).

The changes introduced to sickness benefit were paralleled by early alterations in other parts of the social security system. Once again, in contrast to the view that income maintenance was an area which eluded the radicalism of the

Thatcher era, Atkinson and Micklewright (1989: 125), in their review of changes to benefits for the unemployed during the first two terms of Conservative administration, conclude that, 'the total effect of the Conservative government's action is such that the structure of benefits for the unemployed in 1988 is quite different from that in 1979'. That review suggests thirty eight significant changes to insurance and means-tested benefits for unemployed people during the years 1979–88. The starker examples are found in outright removal of entitlement to benefits which had previously been available, as in the abolition of earnings-related supplements to national insurance unemployment benefit. Less direct changes include the introduction of charges, such as those for postal claimants, and the 'hidden constant' changes, in which the cash value of particular benefits is frozen, thus eroding their purchasing value each year.

Amendments to social security benefits during the first decade of Conservative administration set in train the withdrawal of public responsibility from areas which had previously been assumed to be part of its uncontested remit. In its place, individuals faced with ill-health or unemployment were to be offered far more conditional forms of help and expected to assume a considerably greater share of the responsibility for helping themselves at times of greatest need. The scale of such changes was already considerable. Atkinson and Micklewright (1989: 139ff) conclude their review by attempting an assessment of the actual cash changes for unemployed claimants produced by the different alterations to benefit entitlement. At a conservative estimate they conclude that, between 1979 and 1988, unemployed people had lost a combined total of £510 million, at an average loss of £3.21 a week. These reductions did not fall equally upon all unemployed groups. One in five claimants were estimated to be better off under the 1988 system than the 1979 entitlements. The four out of five who lost, however, included a third of the total number who would have gained more than £4 each week by a return to the former system, with such gainers concentrated among the lower income ranges. In other words, those who could afford to lose the least, had turned out to lose the most.

5.2 The Fowler Reviews

The early attempts at social security reform, although substantial in aggregate, were relatively piecemeal in conception. This period came to an end with the announcement, in 1985, of the Reviews instigated by Norman Fowler, then Secretary of State for Social Security. The Reviews were headlined by government as a root-and-branch investigation of the welfare state, which was to reform, refurbish and re-equip the Beveridge inheritance for a new century. The DHSS characterised the process as one which would lead to 'the most important changes in the safety net of support provided by the state since the 1930s' (Becker 1997: 65). Behind the fine words lay a series of purposes which Bradshaw (1992: 83) summarises as 'privatisation, selectivity, managerialism, incentives and last, but certainly not least, the needs of the economy'. Overlaying the proposals which emerged in the White Paper *The Reform of Social Security: Programme for Action* was what Dean (1993: 86) has characterised as 'an agenda set by right-wing ideologues who wished to see a diminution of Welfare State activity'.

In the words of the White Paper itself, the 'basic principle' which the government set out to reaffirm was that 'social security is not a function of the state alone. It is a partnership between the individual and the state – a system built on twin pillars' (DHSS 1985: para. 1.5). In the practical reforms which followed, however, the weight to be borne by each of the 'twin pillars' was to be amended. In a major reorganisation, supplementary benefits disappeared, to be replaced by Income Support and the range of discretionary additional Single Payments which Supplementary Benefits provided were swept away, to be replaced by the Social Fund. The result was to reduce significantly the amount of help available to the most vulnerable.

The Social Fund

The genesis and practical operation of the Social Fund has been considered at length by a range of social policy commentators (see, for example, Meacher 1985; Cohen and Tarpey 1988; Huby and Walker 1991; Craig 1992; Becker 1997). It is not part of the purpose of this book to rehearse many of the important arguments developed in these texts. However, despite the very small proportion of total social security expenditure which the Fund represents (no more than 0.2 per cent of the total social security budget in 1989/90 according to Cohen *et al.* (1996: 3)), its policy importance means that some consideration needs to be given to those elements which redefine the private and public boundary in relation to those most in need of help from the social security system. In doing so, five different characteristics may be isolated, which marks the Fund out as embodying significant departures in post-war policy in this area.

- The administration of the Fund operates according to the relatively unfettered discretion of local social security officers. In a new departure applicants to the Fund – as they were to be known – were not to be allowed a right of independent appeal against decisions made about claims. While decisions were thus being moved from a public, rule-based scheme to the private determination of state officials, the right of private individuals to challenge decisions made in the name of the public was significantly diminished.
- The system was cash-limited. If the Fund was empty, then no matter how great the need, a payment could not be made. The applicant would be beyond the help of the system.
- Even where payments could be made, the Social Fund shifted the mode of assistance from grants to loans. In future only a minority of payments were to be made by grants. Indeed, Craig (1993: 121) records two contemporary reports from different DHSS offices in a Hertfordshire County Council survey,

where counterclerks told claimants, 'there aren't any grants now, only loans . . . we can't give a grant to anyone in the community unless you can lay your hand on your heart and say they'd be likely to go into an institution tomorrow if we didn't give a grant'.

Individual claimants, paying back loans by direct deduction from benefit, find themselves, as a result, with less to live on each week than the basic scale rates allow. The Social Security Consortium (Ward 1987: 6) concluded that dependence upon the state was to be replaced by 'hidden forms of dependence' on families, friends, charities, money-lenders and loan sharks. Thus, as Oppenheim and Lister (1996: 95) suggest, the Fund had the impact of privatising responsibility, shifting burdens previously undertaken by the state and displacing them onto individuals.

- Finally, the Fund created a category of claimant hitherto unknown in post-war social security policy – the person too poor to be helped. Where an applicant was assessed by Fund officers as deserving of help, but so impoverished as to be unable to repay the loan which might be offered, an offer of help was to be denied. A considerable number of claimants found themselves in this position. In 1991/92, for example, more than 66,000 individuals were so poor as to be excluded from the system designed to alleviate poverty. Craig (1998: 53) estimates that, less than ten years into the Fund's operation, 'cumulatively considerably more than half a million applicants were refused help because of "inability to pay"'. The denial of public responsibility which this policy embodies is the sharpest single example within the general re-drawing of obligations by which the Fund was characterised.

The cumulative effect of these policy changes was to create a system in which losers emerged as a deliberate but unacknowledged effect of policy. Craig (1993: 124) provides a detailed statistical scrutiny which suggests that the cumulative effect of Fund operation has been to create 'a clear and growing division between the ways in which these awards were allocated'. The process of classification is one which divides claimants into the 'deserving' and the 'undeserving' according to circumstance, rather than need.

As unemployment was renewed in the recession of the 1990s, applications to the Fund grew, leading to a change in outcomes. While community care grant applications increased by almost a million, from 269,000 in 1988/90 to 1,266,000 in 1994/95, the proportion of successful applications fell from 52 to 23 per cent (Cohen *et al.* 1996). This radical reduction in the prospects of success from the Fund was not due to a change in the characteristics of claimants. Rather, the rationing process simply became more and more restrictive as demands for help grew. In the process, the stigma and diminishing likelihood of success acted to deter some applicants altogether. Certainly, from the official evaluation of the Fund, it was apparent that the difference between claimants and non-claimants did not lie in the circumstances of the two groups, the researchers concluding that 'there was nothing to distinguish the needs of those who received them from those who did not' (Huby and Dix 1992). As Craig (1998: 53) suggests, one of the privatising measures associated with the Fund has been the way in which the hidden need of those deterred from making an application has obscured from public consciousness the 'extent of poverty created, but hidden, by the social fund'.

Thus, at a time when absolute incomes of the poorest were in decline (Hills 1997), the social welfare system most designed to attend to that poverty had altered as well, removing help which had previously been available and privatising the consequences. The concluding verdict upon the social fund might be left to Craig and Dowler (1997: 117) who characterise it as 'the most extreme example of the government's determination to "privatise poverty"'.

Young people and benefits

This account of privatisation and social security during the middle years of Conservative administration would not be complete without some consideration of the changes which were brought about in the benefit treatment of young people. The collapse of paid employment for young people leaving school at the end of compulsory education is one of the most striking phenomena to be traced in the social circumstances of those generations entering the labour market during the last quarter of the twentieth century (see Haines and Drakeford 1998 for a fuller discussion). In 1976, the year before the introduction of the first Youth Opportunities Programme, 53 per cent of young people went directly into employment at the end of formal schooling. By 1986, ten years later, the proportion had fallen to 15 per cent. As a result, and despite a plethora of make-work training schemes, unemployment among young people persisted. The Government's response, in 1988, was to abolish benefit entitlement for 16- and 17-year-olds.

It was a scandal, Ministers argued, that young people should be afforded the morally sapping choice of living off the largess of the state when a place upon a Youth Training Scheme could be guaranteed to anyone unable to find a 'real' job or continue in education. Entitlement to benefit was withdrawn, as a consequence. Underpinning this removal of young people from the benefit system was a belief in the private responsibility which ought to be assumed for their care and maintenance. Young people, it was claimed, ought to be living at home and looked after by their parents. Moreover, not only 16 and 17 years olds were meant to be in this position. Those young people aged between 18 and 24 were transferred to a new restricted level of benefit on the basis that these, too, ought to be living at home. In fact, as Craig (1998: 55) establishes, 'only 43% of women and 63% of men still lived with their parents by the time they were 21'. The practical effect of these changes has already been noted in Chapter 4. The market reacted by denying access to scarce supply of accommodation to the newly impoverished sources of demand. Once again, responsibility for dealing with these changes was to lie where it fell, in the lives of those concerned.

5.3 Peter Lilley and 'sectoral reform'

The Fowler reforms, which were to have equipped the social security system for a new millennium, lasted for a single parliament. The return of a Conservative government again in 1992 brought a new Secretary of State for Social Security and a new approach to benefit reform. If social security had, indeed, occupied a relatively lowly place in the Thatcherite project, Alcock (1997: 24) suggests that the area now became the one in which the administration of the new Prime Minister, John Major, most sought to develop the New Right agenda. Under the direction of Peter Lilley – the minister who, more than any other, 'might have been expected to ensure that there should be "no turning back"' (Alcock 1997: 25) – the 'big bang' approach of the 1988 changes was abandoned in favour of a 'sectoral' strategy in which different elements within the benefit system were to be tackled in turn. The basis of the approach was a combination of the long-standing Conservative belief that contemporary levels of social security expenditure were economically unsustainable, coupled with a more recent neo-liberal assertion that the social consequences of benefit dependency were so problematic in themselves that the system had become a cause of difficulty in its own right. According to the estimates of the DSS, the sector-by-sector approach was expected to have 'taken some £5 billion a year out of the social security budget by the year 2000' (DSS 1995). The advantages of sectoral reform were to be found both in the greater concentration it allowed upon individual aspects of the system, and the fact that piece-by-piece reform tended to limit objections to the group most directly affected at any one time, thus obscuring the cumulative impact of cut-backs. In the words of Ruth Lister (1996), it amounted to a strategy of 'permanent revolution'.

Taken together, the reforms of the Lilley period were more substantial and significant than those of 1988. Following Becker (1997) the most important can be identified as: the introduction of the Child Support Agency in 1993; the radical restructuring of social security arrangements for community care and residential care in 1993; the reform of invalidity benefits in 1995 and of housing benefit (including restricted help with mortgage costs – see Chapter 4) during 1995/96; the abolition of unemployment benefit and its replacement by the job-seekers allowance in 1996; the additional restriction of benefits for asylum seekers and young people under 25 in 1996; and the further reform of statutory sick pay in the last year of the Conservative administration, 1997.

Considerations of space do not allow a detailed consideration of each of these initiatives. However, an analysis may be built up by using the categories which Lilley himself provided in his Mais lecture of 1993, outlining a series of ways in which, in addition to further means-testing, reform could be brought about. These included: categorisation (e.g. raising the retirement age for women to sixty five), defining need more narrowly (e.g. limiting incapacity benefit through a change in the definition of incapacity), tighter enforcement (e.g. the rules for Restart), conditionality (e.g. the new job-seekers agreement) and contributions tests (tightened up considerably for unemployment benefit). In terms of the issues with which this book is most closely concerned, of course, each of these strategies is linked by the effort to redraw the boundary between the responsibility of the state and of the individual. Lilley expressed this unambiguously in the same lecture when declaring that: 'There is no escaping the need for structural reforms of the social security system. Any effective structural reforms must involve either better targeting or more self-provision, or both.'

Better targeting and self-provision are comfortable words for some very uncomfortable changes. One example must suffice to illustrate the extent to which the state withdrew, during this period, from responsibilities which it had uncontentiously accepted for fifty years or more – the replacement of Income Support and Unemployment Benefit with the Job Seekers Allowance (JSA).

In a number of instances the JSA represented an extension of, rather than a new departure in, social security policy. It embodied many of the techniques which Peter Lilley had described in his Mais lecture. The contribution conditions of unemployment benefit were unilaterally amended so that instead of national insurance payments guaranteeing twelve months benefit, the period was reduced to six. Categorisation changes were applied again to 18–24 year-olds for whom unemployment benefit was to be paid at a reduced rate, even though contribution conditions would have remained as for older claimants. New and more onerous 'availability' and 'actively seeking work' requirements made the conditionality of the benefit harder to meet. In all these aspects, the JSA represents what Silburn (1992: 139) identifies as the 'privatisation of risk', in relation to unemployment and job insecurity. At a time, as he suggests, when labour market changes are producing patterns of instability, 'even amongst those who traditionally have thought of themselves as economically and socially secure', the state has engaged in a withdrawal from the assistance needed in these circumstances.

As well as carrying former policies further, the Job Seekers Allowance also moved the general effort to reduce state responsibility into new territory. The already fragile nature of voluntary participation in state-determined job hunting was overturned by a compulsory scheme in which benefit disqualification was the price for default. Employment advisers were also equipped with new powers to require claimants to engage in particular activities, or desist from others, provided – in the opinion of the adviser – such a Direction would improve the prospects of an individual obtaining work. Once again, refusal to comply with such a Direction would lead to disqualification. It was in the nature of this disqualification, however, that the JSA was innovative. Since 1979 successive Conservative administrations had extended the level of penalty which unemployed people faced, if failing to comply with tightening eligibility criteria. The first Thatcher administration extended the disqualification period from 6 weeks to 13. Eighteen months later the period was extended again to 26 weeks. Atkinson and Micklewright (1989: 128–9) draw out the significance of these changes in this way:

'The more than four-fold increase in the maximum disqualification period from NI benefit (and reduction in SB) in the case of voluntary quitting, industrial misconduct or refusal of a job offer, has changed a parameter of the benefit system that had been in operation for much of the century: the original 1911 Act, the two major inter-war Acts of 1920 and 1934, and the post-Beveridge 1946 Act all stipulated a six-week figure.'

The Government's own Social Security Advisory Committee (1988: 14) also expressed substantial caveats in relation to the extension of disqualification to 26 weeks:

'Disqualification from unemployment benefit for six months, with reduced income support entitlement, is a harsh penalty and one which should therefore be applied with care. We regret that voluntary unemployment is an area in which claimants may be assumed "guilty" until they can prove their "innocence" in that where the benefit officer suspects voluntary unemployment he or she may suspend payment of benefit pending a decision by the adjudication officer on disqualification.'

The JSA changes carried this process one step further. Claimants who are suspended from benefit are denied any help at all, even at the reduced rate, for an initial period of two weeks, unless it can be established that another member of the claimant's household would suffer hardship as a result. This rule means that single people will automatically be left without benefit altogether. Further infringement of the rules leads to longer periods of disqualification, again without any means of support. In the year ending March 1994, 145,094 unemployed claimants were disqualified from benefit. In the same year, a further 181,998 individuals were eventually found to have been suspended in error and benefit restored. Under the JSA changes, many of these would have found themselves without any income from the benefit system through which their most basic needs might be met. Social security, it has been suggested, 'has become the policy ambulance to pick up and deal with all the casualties of the new economic order' (Evans 1997: 94). Some JSA casualties have been driven over by the ambulance itself.

Becker (1997: 77) suggests that, in this period, 'some of the earlier "radical" proposals for social security restructuring from groups such as Conservative Way Forward and the Adam Smith Institute had finally been implemented'. The tests which Peter Lilley had set as rationales for this radicalism were better targeting on the one hand, and greater self-provision on the other. Detailed analysis by David Piachaud (1996) has revealed that better targeting has not been achieved by such strategies. The bottom two quintiles of the population – that is to say, those where a targeting approach would most have concentrated help – together received 63 per cent of cash benefits in 1979. By 1993 this had fallen to 59 per cent. Self-provision, by contrast, had been forcibly extended to those for whom the state no longer made provision, even at times of acute need. This chapter now turns to a social security area where the active promotion of more voluntary self-provision became a key policy of government during the 1980s and early 1990s – that of personal pensions.

5.4 Personal pensions

Waine's (1995: 318) account of the personal pension policies developed by government during the late 1980s and early 1990s begins by linking their genesis to the rise of radical right and neo-liberal thinking within the Conservative Party. Mrs Thatcher's favourite economist, Hayek, was a long-standing opponent of state pension systems, regarding them as an unwarranted intrusion upon personal liberty to determine income in old age (Hayek 1960). Individual ownership of pension arrangements would both promote freedom, and bring with it the other Schumpeterian benefits – responsibility, enterprise and economy.

Waine (1995: 322) describes personal pensions as 'contribution schemes with no set relationship between the pension on retirement and earnings at work, rather returns are based on contributions and the investment performance of the plan'. Collective schemes, such as occupational pensions or the State Earnings Related Pension Scheme (SERPS), are characterised by guaranteed levels of income in retirement, albeit ones over which the individual has no real form of influence. Personal pensions, by contrast, were founded by an individualistic principle, in which self-interested economic actors would seek out the best deal for themselves in a market characterised by competition and variety of supply. While the guarantees of collective provision would be missing, the compensating rewards, in terms of choice and final outcome, would be more than adequate compensation. As Fawcett (1995: 163) makes clear, however, 'the key point is that even to contemplate such a move [the abolition of SERPS] the Conservatives needed a large and advanced private pension industry. In contrast to other areas, such as private health insurance, the industry was already well established.'

The potential flaw in this arrangement was highlighted in response to the Green Paper produced as part of the Fowler reviews. Criticism centred, as Waine (1995: 323) suggests, upon the 'possible disjuncture between ideological concerns with ownership and the adequacy of benefits provided by personal pensions'. The CBI questioned the sense of relying for security in old age upon the 'individual speculative investments' which personal pensions represented. The industry itself was also sceptical. Waine quotes the formal response to the Green Paper of Reed Stenhouse Financial Services: 'we accept that the proposals will give personal freedom to the consumer – they will certainly not give value for money to the consumer.'

The White Paper which followed – *Reform of Social Security: Programme for Action* – made a number of concessions to these concerns, including the modified retention of SERPS, which had originally been proposed for abolition. The financial risks to individuals taking out, or transferring, to personal pensions were to be ameliorated by an incentive financed from the National Insurance Fund in order to encourage people 'to start saving for their own pension' (White Paper, para. 2.30).

The response to this campaign of encouragement was very positive. The Department of Social Security had originally estimated that some half a million people would 'opt out' of SERPS or an occupational pension, in favour of the new personal variety (National Audit Office 1990, para. 3.18). In fact, by the end of 1992/93, five million people had made personal pension arrangements (DSS 1994: 9). According to Fawcett (1995: 163–4), 'the furore was reminiscent of the excitement generated by the industrial privatisations of the early 1980s' in which the financial incentives provided by government 'created the over-heated atmosphere of a limited special offer'.

Hubris, however, was close at hand. The National Insurance incentive which the Secretary of State had justified as helping to 'get the ball rolling' at a minimal cost of some £60 million was soon rolling out of control. Personal pensions were intended to save public money, as self-provision replaced the provision of the state. In fact, as Waine (1995: 328) suggests, the estimated cost of tax reliefs on contributions to personal pensions and the National Insurance incentives during 1987–93 were £7.2 billion and £2.5 billion respectively, pro-viding a total cost to the public purse of £9.7 billion. Pensions bought in this fashion may be 'private', but they are certainly far from being free of depend-ence upon the state.

Most notoriously, however, the vision of competent and confident individual economic actors, successfully pursuing their own best interests, was badly dam-aged by a series of scandals in which it emerged that large numbers of people had been attracted into leaving the security of occupational schemes for the illusory benefits of a personal pension. Hard-selling and misleading advice com-bined to overwhelm even the most determined individual. Self-regulation proved inadequate in containing the errors promulgated by sales agents of the most respected companies. As a result, thousands of individuals were left with a form of self-provision which was either worse than the benefits which had been available under their collective schemes or entirely useless as payments could not be maintained and all contributions were swallowed up by high rates of sales commission. Within this general picture, particular groups in the commun-ity were especially badly affected. Waine (1995: 327) shows a clear picture, drawn from statistical analysis, 'of a financial product having been sold over-whelmingly to people on low incomes'. Others, such as Land and Ward, con-firmed their earlier predictions (1985: 42) that personal pensions would 'be poor value for women, [and] may carry substantial risks for them'.

The ambitions which the privatisers and marketeers brought to the benefit system were thus a good deal less successful in practice than their promoters had suggested, as the Social Security Advisory Committee concluded [*document 7*]. Where the state possessed draconian powers, as in the case of young people and the Job Seekers Allowance, cuts were possible and government felt able, for the most part, to distance itself from the consequences. Faced with a more powerful political lobby, as in the case of pensioners, a different course of action followed. Those already best placed to help themselves were assisted to maxim-ise that advantage. For those left dependent upon a withering state pension, the ground had been cleared for what Sullivan (1996: 31) suggests as an ultimate ambition to 'rid government of responsibility for older people'.

The reform of individual benefits, and the changing nature of responsibility between individual and the state, was underpinned during this period by changes in the administrative apparatus of social security. The combination of these different privatising strands are best demonstrated by the introduction of the Child Support Agency to which this chapter now turns.

5.5 Child Support Agency and the Next Steps initiative

This consideration of privatisation and marketisation in relation to social security has, for the most part, concentrated upon the income maintenance services and systems directly operated by the state. In considering the Child Support Agency, however, a new set of considerations have to be introduced because, as the name implies, the child support system introduced in 1993 found its structural location within a new framework, very different to that of a traditional government department. This new structure is of interest to this book because it forms part of a wider thrust to alter the nature of government, which was consistent, as Greer (1994: 7) suggests, with the 'private good, public bad' dichotomy which was so pervasive a characteristic of policy making during the Conservative period.

The Next Steps agencies, of which the Child Support Agency is among the most prominent, found their origin in a thirty-page report, *Improving Management in Government: the Next Steps* (Jenkins *et al.* 1988). Greer (1994: 6) describes this as 'glossy, bold and evangelical' and 'more like a report from a management consultancy firm than a traditional civil service review'. The document suggested a radical new approach to the business of government in which the work of traditional departments was to be assessed according to a set of new criteria derived from a combination of the public choice theories and new public management discussed in Chapter 2. The Centre for Public Services (1997: 12) describes the process of assessment as a hierarchical one, in which the following tests were to be applied, in turn:

a. Abolition: must the public sector be responsible for the function; can it be abolished or dispersed within government?
b. Privatisation: must the public sector provide the function itself; if not, what form of privatisation is feasible?
c. Strategic contracting out i.e. competitive tendering without an in-house bid.
d. Market testing i.e. competitive tendering with in-house bids.
e. Rationalisation or merger with other agencies.

Any function of government could only be considered at a higher point on the scale if it could not be satisfactorily resolved at an earlier stage. Next Steps agencies, from the outset, occupied a potentially ambiguous position between privatisation and market testing. In practice, Next Steps agency staff remained employed as civil servants, Ministers retained responsibility for overall policy and assessment of performance, while agency management were left free to manage the implementation and delivery of policy. This distinction, in which accountability (which cannot be delegated) was separated from responsibility (which can), largely failed to gain credibility outside the circles where it had been devised.

The Next Steps initiative obtained a remarkably swift hold over government policy. The agency model was proposed and accepted in 1988 and within a year the first agencies were established. Nowhere was action swifter than in the Department of Social Security where, as Greer (1994: 32) suggests, 'the transformation of the department as a result of the Next Steps has been extraordinarily dramatic'. Within five years, the whole Department had been divided into six agencies, covering 97 per cent of all Social Security staff, 68,000 of whom were employed by the Benefit Agency alone. Agency status was intended to confer the usual neo-liberal benefits of cost saving, efficient operation and sensitivity to customer needs. The Centre for Public Services (1997: 20) suggests that the actual outcome was less advantageous than the claims. In a detailed analysis of Social Security agency expenditure between 1990/91 and 1995/96 for example, it concludes that 'administrative costs as a percentage of benefit expenditure has remained virtually static . . . claims about reduced running costs clearly do not apply to several agencies at the core of the British welfare state'.

In terms of the focus of this book, two features of the Child Support policy are of particular relevance. Firstly, it represented a further effort to re-allocate responsibility between the state and the individual. A leaked Cabinet discussion document which set the scene for the new arrangements contained a list of proposals in relation to lone parents and benefits which included 'cuts in benefits for lone parent claimants who have another child, make grandparents responsible for teenage mothers, require lone parents to sign on when their children reach a certain age, and change homelessness legislation to remove the priority status of lone parents (Garnham and Knights 1994: 8). Yet, in all the difficulties which the Agency has faced, few have dissented from the principle which Mrs Thatcher set out as the basis for reform: 'No father should be able to escape from his responsibility' (speech to the National Children's Homes, 17 January 1990). In practice, the extension of state intrusion into private lives in order to secure this principle is one of the paradoxes of privatisation. In the attempt to free itself of the economic burden of paying for children, public officials have acquired powers of intervention into the lives of mothers (with significant benefit penalties for those who fail to comply) which seem far from a determination to roll back the frontiers of the state. Secondly, the nature of Agency status has meant that responsibility for the day-to-day implementation of the policy has been removed from direct public scrutiny. Questions to Ministers are routinely referred to Agency Chief Executives rather than receiving replies for which the policy makers might be held accountable. The boundary between public scrutiny and administrative privacy has been altered in the process.

In common with almost all the policy areas considered in this text, the reform of social security administration continued until the end of the Conservative period in office. Pressure for additional cuts in expenditure led, in 1996, to the announcement of the 'Change Programme', which aimed to reduce operating costs within the DSS by a quarter *[document 9]*. This drastic target was to be reached by a combination of measures including the removal of significant rights to independent appeal against benefit decisions, the abolition of the freephone benefits helpline, the removal of the emergency out-of-hours service used primarily by people facing an immediate emergency or crisis, and a large-scale closure programme of smaller Benefit Agency offices. A number of elements in this programme had already been implemented by the May General Election of 1997. In Becker's (1997: 85) summation the plans were consistent with the government's reforms in health and social care, 'internal markets and the greater use of the private sector in administering benefits – in effect the privatisation of the delivery of benefits'. Nor did plans end there. The right wing Conservative MPs in the No Turning Back Group (1993) were already on record as suggesting that self-provision could be extended much further, with the state withdrawing from basic benefits such as the old age pension, unemployment and disability benefits.

5.6 Privatisation, social security and the individual

The argument of this chapter has been one which suggests that, while the dominant metaphor which British social policy applies to the welfare state is that of the 'safety net', the threadbare and inadequate condition of the sanctuary which it provides, means that the metaphor has come to cast a misleading light upon the development of recent welfare policy. The reliance upon the market and an active redrawing of the rules of entitlement, in favour of self-provision, have provided the main policy thrusts of recent times. The social security system which results, and which has been set out here, is no longer one which fails to help through neglect or accident, but one which proceeds through a deliberate targeting of certain individuals to place them beyond the safety net.

This chapter ends with an attempt to demonstrate these techniques in action through an investigation of the help which poorest citizens might receive at a time of acute need – that of death and bereavement. The welfare state famously began with a commitment to promote and protect the well-being of its citizens 'from the cradle to the grave'. Beveridge (1942: 151) put it simply *[document 1]*: 'All people when they die need a funeral.' In a single sentence summary of the Social Insurance and Allied Services Report, funeral costs were explicitly included. The public were to be offered 'a scheme of social insurance against interruption and destruction of earning power and for special expenditure arising at birth, marriage and death'. The taint of a pauper's grave was thus to be removed through social insurance. Provision would be universally and unequivocally made for the costs of a decent burial.

The state of provision today is very different. Changes in social security, and the impact which this has on other social systems, have radically diminished the protections on offer and the security which those dependent upon the system can expect. The universal Death Grant was abolished soon after the Conservatives came to office in 1979. Reformed arrangements were introduced with the Social Fund which retained only three circumstances through which a claimant could look for an automatic, as-of-right, payment. These were cold weather payments, a maternity grant and a payment to meet the costs of a funeral. Despite the general context of cut-back and deterrence, therefore, the specific identification of benefits for this purpose illustrates the continuing force which the twin poles of cradle and grave continued to exercise over policy makers. Even when other payments were so fiercely under attack, the basic decencies of ensuring help at the time of greatest vulnerability, of birth and death, remained embedded within the system.

Despite the deterrent nature of the Fund, the onset of a fresh economic recession in the years immediately after its introduction served to force up the numbers of people obliged to make claims to it. In 1988/89 40,000 individuals were given help with funeral expenses from the Fund, at a cost of £18 million. In 1991 about 50,000 claims were made and awarded. Just under £30 million was paid out at a rough average of £600 per claim. By 1993/94 the numbers had risen to 72,000 and the payments to £63 million. The average award had risen to £924.

As in the case of Severe Hardship payments for young people, discussed earlier, the system under which such help was delivered had been devised entirely by government. It is at least perverse, therefore, to find the same government attacking the rules which they themselves had established. It was in just this way that help with funeral expenses came under attack from Peter Lilley at the end of November 1994. He told the House of Commons that:

'I shall be limiting the grant paid through the social fund for funeral payments. Levels of payments for funerals through the social fund have grown by 6 per cent a year above inflation. Funeral payments cover the whole cost, so funeral directors can force up costs to customers on social fund, knowing that they are unlikely to obtain better quotes.' (Peter Lilley MP, *Hansard* H.C., Vol. 125, col. 1208, 30 November 1994)

The Social Security Advisory Committee (1995) once again objected to the draft regulations:

'We have been presented with no evidence that a simple but dignified and respectful funeral could be provided universally in the United Kingdom for £875 or less. In many areas the cost would be considerably higher and a national ceiling of £875 will leave a large number of poor people with a considerable shortfall in their funeral bills.'

No account was taken of these views, or those from other sources. By September 1995 the new set of more restrictive rules were being applied to Social Fund Funeral payments. A global maximum of £875 was established as the most that the Fund would pay for all items. The DSS claimed to have reached this figure by averaging out payments over the previous period. In fact, in one of those statistical sleights of hand which had become characteristic of government declarations in social policy areas, the amount paid out had been divided by the total number of claims made – both successful and unsuccessful. The inclusion of those who had received no help at all had the effect of reducing the average amount apparently paid to those who were entitled. The figure thus represented a greater cut in the help which any individual claimant might expect to obtain.

The September 1995 changes attempted to reduce expenditure still further through the introduction of new rules concerning the person 'responsible' for a funeral. Where the deceased had one or more than one close surviving relative a new 'ability to pay' test was to be applied. In a first step, Benefit Agency staff were to establish whether or not the contact of a close relative was equal to, or greater than, that of the claimant. If that question could be answered in the affirmative then the claimant was to be refused a payment provided the other relative was not also in receipt of a qualifying benefit. The actual willingness of that other relative to undertake responsibility for the funeral was not be taken into account.

The combination of the cap on funeral director's expenses and the 'ability to pay' rule produced a reduction in help available from the Fund from £63 million in 1994/95 to £47 million in 1995/96, exceeding government targets for cut-backs. Not only were fewer people receiving help, the average payment to those able to obtain assistance had fallen from £924 to £791. Once again, the target of a reduction to £875 had been exceeded. Expenditure on funeral payments fell by more than 25 per cent between 1994/95 and 1995/96.

Encouraged by this success, the Minister decided to act again. In November 1996, he announced a further series of changes to funeral payments from the Fund, to take place as from 1 April 1997. A newly lowered ceiling of £600 was to apply, producing a minimum anticipated saving of a further £4 million. At the same time, further changes to the liable relative rule were introduced. Since 1 April 1997, if a relative can be found who is not on benefit, then an application will not be allowed from an individual who is a claimant. Put simply, if the Benefit Agency comes to believe that the costs of a funeral could be laid at the door of a relative who is not eligible for Social Fund help, they will not make any payment to anyone who is eligible. This means, in an example chosen by one national newspaper, that a lone mother would be denied help with the cost of a child's funeral if the father of the child is traceable and not claiming benefit. Commenting on that example, a spokesperson for the DSS said that it would be 'unreasonable' to act otherwise (*The Guardian* 2.11.96).

Once again, the fact that the Benefit Agency are able to identify some other relative who is not a claimant does not mean that any such relation will have to pick up the bill. It simply means that the Benefit Agency will refuse to meet a Social Fund application. The Government estimated that 7,000 people who would have been able to get help in 1996/97 would not be able to get help after April 1997 as a result of these changes.

Individuals who are no longer able to obtain help from the social security system have to look elsewhere for assistance. The Benefit Agency's own advice document (Benefit Agency 1995) includes a paragraph headed in capital letters HELP FROM THE COUNCIL. It says 'the local council has a duty to bury or cremate a dead person if no other arrangements have been made'. These duties arise from the Public Health (Control of Diseases) Act of 1984, which requires a local authority to provide a burial where 'no suitable arrangements for the disposal of the body have been or are being made otherwise than by the Authority' (section 46, subsection 1).

Evidence from Wales (Drakeford 1997b) shows that the help which any individual might obtain in these circumstances is variable, at best. Some local authorities approach this duty with sensitivity, determined to provide a service which has no less dignity or consideration than would be afforded to any other individual. Others report very different responses, including some which would not be out of place in a Dickensian novel: 'They get a pauper's grave, opened to the minimum, with no exclusive right of burial and with no sort of memorial.'

Changes in one social system produce results outside the boundaries of that system itself. The direct impact of alterations in the Social Fund meet a number of other important social policy developments which add to the significance of these changes for local authorities. The new demands which authorities face come not only from individuals left with no other resort, but from changes in patterns of institutional social care. One of the strongest themes in the responses to the survey in Wales was a widespread concern at the increased demand for 1984 Act burials from nursing and residential homes for older people. The separation of 'social' and 'medical' care has moved many such individuals out of hospitals and into the commercial market. 'Care in the community' then means, for many older people, that they end their lives in institutions paid for by the state and without the comfort of relatives or friends (Jack 1991; Harding et al. 1996). Reports received from council officers contained accounts in which the commercial sector reacted to death in these circumstances as though left with a product which had ceased to be an asset, and determined to write off that loss as soon as it could be shifted to someone else's account. More than one authority reported being telephoned by residential homes before death of an elderly resident had taken place, with pressure applied to make arrangements for removal on the grounds that a bed could thus be released for a new and paying customer.

Further evidence of the pressures caused in such circumstances arose in the summer of 1998 when the local government Ombudsman for the North of England published a highly critical report of the actions of Castle Morpeth Council in Northumberland. Here, the local authority had, during the summer of 1997, informed care homes within its area that it would not accept responsibility for the burial of former residents under the 1984 Public Health Act provisions. A letter to establishments made the council's position clear: 'A residential home is the last home for many people, and, just as you would provide for their needs when they arrive, so you should provide for their needs when they depart.' The policy change came to a head over an individual case when an elderly woman, who had no known relative and very few assets, died at a home within the authority's boundary. The council refused to accept responsibility for burial. When the home complained to the Ombudsman, the local authority defended its position explicitly in the terms of the new privatised market. It wrote to the Ombudsman: 'One could argue that from a commercial view point residents of a home are its income-producing raw material. Ergo, from a purely commercial view, deceased residents may then be regarded as being waste produced by their business.' Patricia Thomas, the Ombudsman for the North of England, rejected this argument as 'far-fetched and insulting'. She ordered the council to meet the costs incurred by the home and to pay compensation to the home owner for the time and trouble which had been incurred.

Whatever the rights and wrongs of the Morpeth case, the general conclusion that the provisions of the 1984 Act are not a safety net seems inescapable. In the terms adopted in this book, individuals denied help by the social security system and forced to look for help elsewhere do not only find themselves beyond the safety net, in the sense that the framework of state provision has been withdrawn from them. The courses of action which they then have to pursue in order to repair that loss, are themselves likely to increase the fragility of their hold on social stability.

The help which is available in relation to funeral expenses from the social security system has been progressively eroded over the past ten years. Both in terms of cash and in terms of eligibility, the scope of assistance has shrunk to the point where the famous promise of the welfare state must surely be regarded as broken. In the argument suggested here, these changes have not occurred as a result of accidental fraying of the safety net. Rather, particular categories of individual have been knowingly and deliberately removed from the scope of assistance. Individuals are left, at great personal cost, to carry the burden which previously had been shared communally through the provision of the welfare state.

5.7 Summary

Social security, as Adrian Sinfield has suggested (1991: 2) is 'primarily a condition not a provision, an end not a means'. The account provided in this chapter has attempted to show, however, some of the ways in which changes in the means have an impact upon the ends. The redrawing of boundaries between the state and the individual, in enhancing choice for some, has had the effect of reducing security for those who are least able to protect themselves. In comparison with 1979, the social security system of 1997 showed the effects of privatisation and marketisation in almost all its dimensions. At an administrative level, services were now provided by agencies which stood at arm's-length from the public sector and which were internally organised along the lines of the new managerialism. The emphasis upon private provision for income at times of need had, for those who could afford it, altered the landscape in relation to pensions and other areas such as housing costs and periods of unemployment.

For those who were left to depend upon the state, the benefits system itself had, in a whole series of different ways, become less generous. While poverty had increased, the help available to deal with its consequences had been reduced. While the application of privatisation in the income maintenance field had proceeded without much of the flag-waving which was so characteristic of the industrial sphere, its social policy implications were profound.

Chapter 6

EDUCATION

The impact of privatisation and marketisation upon education policy during the Conservative years after 1979 was profound. Yet, compared to the industrial field, where explicit and celebratory references to privatisation were so characteristic, the application of such policies in education was far less overt. Indeed, Flude and Hammer (1990: 68) suggested that 'public rhetoric from government spokespersons has tended to avoid the terms "privatisation" when referring to education, unlike statements on many other publicly provided services'. Despite this reticence, however, in education, as in other social policy dimensions, the boundary between public and private provision was shifting in a series of ways, driven largely by the influence of those who believed in the benefits to be gained from a diminution in the role of publicly organised and provided services and their substitution by private provision and private choice.

Three different strands can be identified in the policy proposals and actions from 1979 onwards. The least recognised approach, but one which had a real impact in relatively limited spheres, may be found in the direct transfer of communally-owned assets to organisations outside the control of the public or their democratic structures. This chapter will deal with this strategy in relation to Grant-Maintained Schools. The second strand, and a more important one, is to be found in what Hargreaves and Reynolds (1989) call 'the increasing privatisation of the financial means for purchasing or gaining access to good quality education'. Consideration of the design and implementation of the Assisted Places Scheme will provide an example of this strategy in action. Thirdly, and most significantly of all, policy in this area during the latter part of the 1980s and the 1990s came to be shaped by the privatisation of decision making. A market in school places was created in which 'providers' – that is to say, schools – were to be removed from the direct control of local education authorities and encouraged to compete for 'purchasers' of their service – that is to say, parents and pupils – in order to survive. The institution of local financial management, in which budgets were devolved to schools through a formula driven by age-weighted pupil numbers, meant that 'purchasers' had real money attached to them through which their market choices might be rendered effective. By the end of the period with which this chapter is concerned, as Taylor-Gooby (1993: 102) argues, there had been a remodelling in 'virtually every aspect of education policy in the UK', as a result of which 'the new education settlement represents the most substantial change in what is taught, to whom and under whose control for half a century'.

This chapter is organised along broadly chronological lines. In doing so, the claims of privatisation advocates will be explained, the strength of these concepts assessed in relation to education policy, and the actual performance of the education system during this period tested against the case made by the free marketeers at the outset. The main ingredients in the neo-liberal case, in terms both of analysis and prescription, have already been set out in the first chapter of this book. Following Bowe *et al.* (1993: 66), the thinking might be summarised in this way. The problem facing the British education system at the onset of the 1980s rested upon schools which depended inertly upon the state, a bureaucratic form of administration which stifled initiative and enterprise, and an education establishment which was complacent and unresponsive to the views of those outside its own charmed circle and which had organised an effective 'producer capture' of a system which now served the interests of whose who worked within it, rather than those who financed or used it. The whole system required reform so as to provide new impetus to the positive values of self-help and self-sufficiency, responsiveness to users and dedicated to quality services delivered in the most cost-effective manner. The mechanisms for achieving this reform were to be found in the strategies and techniques of free markets and privatisation. Their application to education was summed up by the influential American school choice theorists, Chubb and Moe (1990: 25) in their argument that:

> 'Control by democratic institutions promotes ineffective organisation and limits autonomy, essentially constraining the ability of schools to respond appropriately to the educational demands of their clientele . . . (so that) if public schools were freed from democratic control and bureaucratic constraints, and instead regulated by the market, they could repeat the success of private schools.'

An investigation and assessment of the practical measures through which such reforms were pursued now follows.

6.1 Early days

Assisted Places Scheme

The most significant early reforms of the Thatcher administration were contained in the 1980 (No. 2) Education Act which aimed to increase the influence of parents in the school system by increasing the amount of information available to them, providing for a limited discretion in choosing schools and additional representation on governing bodies. It established the Assisted Places Scheme, which held out the prospect of the children of low-income families attending schools in the private sector free of charge or at a reduced rate. The scheme clearly embodied a privatising agenda, in its transfer of money directly into the private, rather than public sphere of education, endorsing the notion that a private education was qualitatively better than anything to be found in the maintained sector. As well as being of symbolic value, the financial impact upon the private sector was considerable. Edwards and Whitty (1997: 33) suggest that, 'for the schools themselves, especially those (almost eighty of them) allocated twenty-five or more places a year, the Scheme makes possible a more academically selective entry than reliance on fee-paying would produce . . . there are now schools with 40 per cent and more of their pupils on assisted places.'

Privatisation through the Assisted Places Scheme was justified primarily on the positive impact it would produce among those whose intellectual abilities were held back by financial and social disadvantage. In practice, research reported by Smith and Noble (1995) has shown that less than 10 per cent of students funded through the APS come from families of manual workers, and one-third of scholarship recipients were at private schools before receiving a state bursary. Whatever reservations might have been established during the life-time of the scheme, however, the political imperatives by which it was surrounded remained powerful throughout the years of Conservative administration. As late as November 1995 the Budget contained an announcement of the doubling in size of the scheme and its extension to children of primary school age (Glennerster 1996: 132).

City Technology Colleges

The Assisted Places Scheme was followed, in 1986, by the development of City Technology Colleges (CTCs), institutions which were to be independent of the local authority and where 'all or a substantial part of the capital costs would be met by private sponsorship' (DES 1986: 8). The colleges were intended to provide choice for parents where existing provision was unpopular or inadequate. Located in areas where the rolls of other schools were falling, they were also to contribute to the raising of standards generally through market mechanisms. The threat of losing able and motivated students, and the money which went with them, was to act as a spur to other institutions to make themselves more attractive to potential students and their parents.

Organisationally, as Edwards et al. (1994: 154) suggest, 'Although they charge no fees, CTCs are organisationally much closer to private than to maintained schools, including the more limited representation given to parents and the non-participation of teachers on their governing bodies.' In terms of the first category of privatisation identified at the start of this chapter, CTCs involved both the direct transfer of public assets to the new sector, and the direct spending of new public money upon them. Once transferred to the colleges themselves, neither the local ratepayers, from whose resources land and buildings had originally been obtained, nor the taxpayers from whom the new allocations had been forthcoming, were able to exercise any form of ownership or control. The initiative undoubtedly drew upon the general willingness of the government to place public assets in private hands, although in this case – unlike the industrial privatisations – it was prepared to do so without any compensation through sale.

In practice, the major importance of CTCs lay, as Edwards *et al.* (1994: 144) suggest, 'in its potential contribution to challenging "monolithic" public provision, blurring the boundary between "public" and "private"'. It thus provided a model for how schools are intended to operate in a new market-orientated system. In practice, the market system has turned out to be rather different from the neutral, choice-promoting, equity-enhancing, mechanism suggested by supporters of the reforms. The relatively lavish resources poured into CTCs, especially when compared with the cash-starved local authority schools in the same areas, soon began to influence the playing field between them. Edwards and Whitty (1997: 38) summarise this aspect of the CTC experiment as 'vigorously promoted and preferentially funded, they can be regarded as a direct intervention in the market, an "interference" in the interplay of supply and demand which has not yet done much to break the mould'.

While the colleges were expected to reflect the nature of their catchment areas, once demand for places at them exceeded supply, a form of selection and rationing of places had to be instituted. Written tests for potential pupils and interviews for potential parents soon created a situation in which, far from customers choosing suppliers, the supplier was able to choose its customers, a strategy which Flude and Hammer (1990: 65), among others, describe as 'selection by stealth'.

Despite these criticisms, both schemes retained a highly regarded place in the official history of education policy during this era. The 1992 White Paper, *Choice and Diversity*, identified and hailed the creation of CTCs which, together with the Assisted Places Scheme, represented 'one of the first significant steps towards an education system characterised by 'choice and diversity' (DfE 1992). As this chapter now turns to the next phase of reform – the 1988 Education Reform Act – the final verdict upon these earlier examples might be left with Dale (1989) who characterised CTCs as 'the most representative emblem' of a broad strategy of 'conservative modernisation'. Briefly, it had become a policy of simultaneously 'freeing' individuals for economic purposes while controlling them for social purposes. The type of education privileged in the reforms was of a firmly traditional variety, delivered either in the private system or within a culture which emphatically emphasised the virtues of discipline, hard work and obedience. Market actors able to bring themselves within such definitions were certainly freer to pursue these goals.

6.2 The Education Reform Act 1988

Despite the fact that the leading neo-liberal, Sir Keith Joseph, had been continuously Secretary of State for Education in the period 1981–86, the reforms of the first two Conservative administrations had failed to live up to the ambitions of the more radical liberalisers within the Party. Indeed, Sir Keith himself bemoaned the fact that he had been convinced by officials that his own enthusiasm for vouchers could not be translated into practice (Ribbins and Sherratt 1997: 82).

The reforms of the first part of the 1980s were successful, however, in creating a climate in which more radical action might follow. Taylor-Gooby (1993) describes the context in this way:

'The direct impact of reforms before the 1987 election was limited, although the changes had severely weakened the powers of teachers, local government and central planners to influence policy. . . . The stage was now set for radical reform. . . . Consensus policy making in education was dead and the way was open for a shift to managed markets in the delivery of education.'

With Sir Keith's retirement, the Education portfolio passed to Kenneth Baker and, with him, the political spotlight fell more sharply upon this policy area. The Conservative Party Manifesto of 1987, *The Next Move Forward*, included several pages of specific proposals – a considerable contrast to the document of 1979 when it had occupied only a few lines *[document 4]*. In the summer which followed the third Conservative General Election victory, a series of consultation papers prepared the way for a new Bill which was published in November of that year. It aimed to create a market in education, based on a strategy of freeing up the demand side and differentiating the supply side.

Local management of schools

The demand side – that is to say, pupils and parents seeking school places – was liberalised by requiring schools to admit as many pupils as set in their 1979 standard intake figure – i.e. at the point where numbers on roll in schools were at or near their height. This element of the Act is usually known as 'open enrolment' and was the basis of government claims to have placed a new priority upon parental choice in education. At the same time, the Act required local authorities to devolve increasing proportions of their education budgets directly to schools through a formula which was driven by the number of pupils in attendance. Taylor-Gooby (1993: 111) concludes that the combination 'effectively introduces paperless vouchers into the state sector, without additional funding for expansion or contraction or for transport to the school of one's choice'. As explored more fully below, however, the value of the voucher, being the same for each child of any given age, provided a powerful set of incentives for schools to compete for the least expensive or most able child (Glennerster 1996: 131). Barrow (1998: 73) suggests that the efficiency arguments in favour of schools being able to control their own budgets needs to be balanced by the loss of economy in the wider school system – 'the pooling of risk was hampered and the economies of scale . . . were not exploited as they were formerly'. Reorganisation of school provision to reduce surplus places became more difficult. The rise in school exclusions included a financial component, as schools found that the loss in funding through excluding a pupil 'may be less than the costs imposed by that pupil on the school'. From the outset, therefore, the idea that the newly created market would be economically efficient and purchaser rather than provider-driven was open to question.

Delegation of budgets, as well as transferring powers to parents, was also rooted in the management theory which, in the privatisation approach, was regarded as the best means of altering producer actions in a competitive market. Conditions needed to be created in which schools regarded one another as rivals for the custom of potential pupils and in which parents could substitute a school of choice for the one to which they might be directed by a local education authority. Only in this way would schools be made 'more responsive to parents' needs as well as more effective in meeting them' (DES 1987).

The connection between open enrolment and local management of schools was completed, in the 1988 Act, by the introduction of the National Curriculum – a detailed subject-by-subject prescription which was to be compulsory for state schools. The National Curriculum, and the regime of regular testing which went with it, was to provide the common currency by which schools might be judged and consumers make judgements in the market place. As Miliband (1990: 7) suggests, 'to make markets work, signals are needed to direct the behaviour of market actors'. In the education reforms, 'these signals are to be provided by testing and publication of results. The curriculum is thus fundamentally an "assessment curriculum".'

Bowe *et al.* (1993: 65) draw together the changes of the 1988 Act era, in neo-liberal terms, in this way: 'The educational process becomes the production process, teachers are producers, parents are consumers, knowledge becomes a commodity and the educated student the product, with a minimum specification laid down by the National Curriculum.' This chapter will return to an assessment of these strategies, against the claims made for them, in a later section. At this point, it is important to introduce another main departure which the 1988 Act embodied, the institution of the grant-maintained school.

Grant-maintained schools

Among the large number of radical proposals contained in the 1988 reforms, the proposal to establish a new category of schools, known as grant-maintained (GM), according to Flude and Hammer (1990: 66) 'created the greatest controversy'. On the basis of a simple majority in a parental ballot and with no required minimum proportion of parents taking part in the ballot, a school could, subject to the approval of the Secretary of State, be taken out of the local authority ambit and transferred to newly created Boards of Governors who would, thereafter, be responsible for their organisation and functioning. As in the case of some CTCs, grant-maintained schools involved the transfer of land and property from the local authority to the school's governing body. In privatisation terms, therefore, this represented a direct shift out of public ownership and control. The schools would, as the Act put it, 'opt out' of the mainstream state sector and become, in Mrs Thatcher's phrase 'independent state schools'.

Local councils, and their local taxpayers, were left with the debt charges produced by original purchase of land and construction of buildings. Thereafter, GM schools would be free to dispose of assets gifted to them, without any scope for influence by those still paying the original bills. Barrow (1998: 72) notes the perverse incentives which this arrangement created. In his study, 'one of the schools ordered a large amount of equipment just before opting out. LEAs also had an incentive not to invest in schools which it believed would opt out.'

As in the case of City Technology Colleges, the promotion of GM schools over the following years was to be characterised by highly preferential treatment in terms of revenue and capital expenditure. The 1992 Autumn Financial Statement, for example, showed government plans to devote almost one-third of its total schools capital allocation budgets to projects in the GM sector over the following three years. In the same year, capital grants averaged £102,000 for each grant-maintained school, as against £28,000 for each maintained school (DES 1992: Table 2).

Grant-maintained schools thus embody a series of essential neo-liberal characteristics [document 8b]. Indeed, although usually most closely associated with Kenneth Baker, both the Adam Smith Institute and the hard-line No Turning Back group of Tory MPs have since claimed ownership of the original proposal (Ribbins and Sherratt 1997: 38). The GM initiative was intended to confer the core advantages of choice, diversity and a demonstration of the gains to be made by releasing the combined energies of empowered parental consumers and freed-up entrepreneurial heads and governors. The basis of the controversy referred to earlier by Flude and Hammer was to be found in the same authors' contention that the initiative would 'further blur the boundaries between public and private schooling and widen the scope of the process of privatisation occurring within education'.

More than ten years after the passing of original legislation, it is now possible to reach some verdicts upon the claims made for the grant-maintained strategy. Towards the end of the period Halpin et al. (1997: 60) estimated that there were 'just over 1000 primary and secondary schools in England' which had opted out of LEA control, comprising approximately 10 per cent of the school age population. These schools were concentrated in particular geographical areas especially – and ironically in view of Kenneth Baker's emphasis on GM schools as an escape route from left-wing local Labour councils – those council areas controlled by the Conservatives. Differential formation of GM schools on the basis of geography was by no means neutral in terms of social need. Of 225 schools covered in a survey by Fitz et al. (1993), only 8 per cent (18 schools) were in areas classified as disadvantaged. Using the powers to set their own admission criteria, Smith and Noble (1995: 62) discovered evidence that GM schools were excluding local children in favour of more promising market material from elsewhere. Of the secondary schools opting out in the first wave (that is, up and running by September 1989), 41 per cent had selective admissions policies – compared with the 4 per cent of selective secondary schools in the LEA sector before the grant-maintained policy took effect (Fitz et al. 1993: 10).

Outside formal admission policies, evidence of market-driven selection was also apparent. Taylor-Gooby (1993: 115) suggests that 'There are already indications that some grant-maintained schools are seeking to exclude pupils who do not perform well in examinations, a policy which will enhance the school's test record, but do little for students who are hard to teach.' The rise in school exclusions within a market framework will be dealt with in a later section of this chapter. On counts of both admission and exit, however, the pattern which emerges is one where, far from parents choosing from a range of educational products, producers gear themselves to 'cream skim' those consumers who will be most to their own advantage.

The shift towards selection in grant-maintained schools casts a light upon another of the major claims of the market enthusiasts. Fitz *et al.* (1993: 7) make the important point that GM schools were originally intended to 'demonstrate that educational outcomes could be explained as arising from the managerial benefits associated with self-governance'; that is to say, the difference was to be made, not by money or by explanations rooted in social difference, but in management itself – a key contention of the privatisers. Gillian Sheppard, the last Conservative Secretary of State in an eighteen-year-long line, cited this characteristic as 'the most important benefit of all' which GM status brings:

> 'I perceive in those running GM schools a terrific spirit of entrepreneurialism, of "Well, let's have a bash at this". . . . In other words, a freeing up of all the enthusiasm, the expertise and ability that is there in people. . . . That is why self-government can be so powerful. Rather than waiting for someone else to tell them what to do, it encourages schools to say to themselves: "We could do that. Let's do it. Now".' (Ribbins and Sherratt 1997: 207–23)

A less enthusiastic verdict upon the connection between GM status and effective and efficient leadership was delivered by the Audit Commission while Mrs Sheppard was still in office. It found that GM schools were in need of significant improvement in the management of their finances, with large differences existing between such schools in the way they managed grants from the Government, totalling £1.6 billion. In particular, the report was critical of the role of school governors, finding that 52 of the 89 schools surveyed 'lacked clearly defined or prioritised objectives'.

Despite these reservations, the principal practical impact of GM schools is to be found in what Glatter *et al.* (1997a: 10) discuss in terms of hierarchy. Despite a specific commitment in the 1992 Education White Paper to diversity without hierarchy: 'The Government wants to ensure that there are no tiers of schools within the maintained system but rather parity of esteem between different schools, in order to offer parents a wealth of choice' (DfE/WO 1992: 1.49) – the actual effect of GM and other reforms was to 'reinforce and consolidate the grouping of schools into tiers, starting with prestige public schools and going through grammar, GM, specialist/CTCs and finishing with local authority or "council schools" in deprived areas at the bottom'.

As noted earlier in this chapter, the basis of a market in education had been framed by its theorists as an essentially neutral and technical matter, in which parents would be free to choose from a plethora of different possibilities, laid out on a level playing field. The treatment of GM schools shows just how far the practice of government departed from the theory it had espoused. Far from treating all schools equally, the framework within which choice was to be exercised was one in which certain producers were heavily favoured over others and in which, as a result, certain products were provided with distinct market advantages. The upshot, Bartlett *et al.* (1998: 6) suggest, is that 'the promotion of GM schools is adversely affecting the "sense of community and collegiality" in the education system. By undermining trust relationships, the introduction of competition in education, as in other sectors, is destroying the motivation and creativity of the profession.'

6.3 After the Reform Act

The reform process in education did not end with the 1988 Act. Three further Acts and a series of other initiatives were to follow in the next six years. The Education (Schools) Act 1992 instituted a national system of four-yearly school inspections, leading to the publication of individual school reports. The purpose of publication was to add to the information available to parents through which rational and calculative choices might better be made. The 1993 Education Act established the national Funding Agency for Schools, abolished the requirement for local authorities to have education committees and envisaged further diminution in the role of local education authorities. It also gave new official sanction to selection. Secondary schools were now to be given the powers to select up to 10 per cent of their intakes, with the basis for selection being special aptitude for an area of the curriculum which the school regarded as its particular strength.

Nor were these themes at an end. The final year of the Major Government was dominated by disputes in the education field. The parliamentary session opened with yet a further Education Bill *[document 8c]* designed to increase school selection, allowing grant-maintained schools to select up to half of their pupils by ability or aptitude without any special permission and allowing local authority schools to select one-fifth of their pupils. The Bill also proposed giving more freedom to grant-maintained schools, tightening rules on school discipline, raising standards through testing for five-year-olds, and target-setting for all schools. The proposals were fiercely resisted. The Secondary Heads Association was reported in *The Independent* of 10 October 1996 as not having been so angry about a White Paper for twenty years:

'The proposals for schools to select up to half their pupils were "undemocratic and unfair". Individual schools would be able to select more pupils without reference to the rest of the community. . . . Parents would have to make multiple applications to hedge their bets "entering their child for a variety of selection tests, criteria hurdles and interviews to safeguard against not getting their first choice".'

The selection proposals were 'incoherent, unfair, divisive, cost-ineffective, administratively burdensome and potentially gender biased'.

The Act only reached the statute book in partial form and as a result of considerable horse-trading with the Labour Party opposition in the dying days of the parliamentary session.

Nursery vouchers

Those debates were coloured and shaped by continuing disputes over the Conservatives' final attempt to put into practice the voucher system *[document 8a]*, so strongly favoured by the most convinced neo-liberals within its own ranks. The scheme was announced, on an experimental basis, by the Prime Minister, John Major, during the summer of 1995. *The Independent* newspaper, on 31 October 1996, recorded the views of Edward Lister, leader of the radical right Wandsworth Council, one of only four councils to agree to participate in the experimental period. Vouchers were to stimulate the market to provide both competition, thus raising standards, and new places, perhaps even new schools, to meet demand. The success of vouchers in the nursery field would lead to their extension to the rest of education.

So determined was this optimism that, despite difficulties which emerged early in the experimental period, the scheme – 'little loved and largely unwanted' according to *The Independent* review – was extended to the whole of England and Wales in the following academic year. In February 1997 a voucher, worth a notional £1,100 a year, was distributed to all eligible parents. According to Glennerster (1996: 135), the actual cost of a full-time place in a nursery school in England in 1993/94 was £3,320 and £2,600 for a place in a nursery class of a primary school. The money to be spent on the scheme was largely recovered by central government from the standard spending assessments of local authorities. As a result, as Glennerster (1996: 135) suggests, 'those who currently spend most money on pre-school facilities will have most taken away. . . . The gainers will be those authorities who have spent least in the past and those parents who can afford to spend money educating their child privately who will now have part of the cost defrayed.'

The nursery voucher scheme was to last only one year, before its abolition by the incoming Labour Government of May 1997. Even within that short life, however, its inherent difficulties and drawbacks had become apparent. The scheme was cumbersome to administer and, at its most basic, failed to guarantee a nursery place. The government agency set up to administer the scheme concluded that more than a quarter of four-year-olds in the pilot areas failed to obtain nursery education (*Labour Research* 1997a). The cash requirements of local education authorities, however, meant that once the scheme was in operation schools were driven to recruit actively in the market for four-year-old children. Admission criteria were altered so as to admit children as soon as they turned four, instead of during the term in which they reached their fifth birthday, while class sizes in infant schools expanded in order to attract the new business and so recoup the money which had been removed to fund the scheme. As a result, far from increasing diversity and promoting choice, the practical impact of nursery vouchers was to drive out the provision which had existed in the private, and especially the informal, sector of play groups and nursery provision, in favour of the bulk services of hard-pressed schools. The chief executive of the Pre-School Learning Alliance, Margaret Lochrie, suggested that hundreds of play groups were likely to close, as local authorities 'dashed for the cash' which could be recouped by increasing the numbers in reception classes. The National Children's Bureau (1996), in an independent investigation of the pilot project, suggested that it 'has done more to push four-year olds into starting primary school early than to expand nursery provision'. The director of the NCB's early childhood unit again emphasised the deteriorating quality of experience provided in reception classes – 'where there may be one teacher for 35 children' – as compared to previous arrangements. The criticisms were all rejected by the Secretary of State of the period, Gillian Sheppard.

6.4 Assessing the reforms

Nursery vouchers complete this chapter's chronological consideration of education initiatives during the Conservative years. Attention now turns to investigating, in more detail, the claims which unite the different individual schemes and projects set out above. To recapitulate briefly, the reforms were based upon the introduction of market principles which, adapting Glatter *et al.* (1997b: 138), were claimed to confer the benefits of choice, diversity, competition, self-determination and equity. A consideration of these claims now follows.

The emphasis, by the New Right pamphleteers, upon the importance of public choice is rooted in an essentially economic perspective which regards behaviour as purposive and based upon careful calculation of rational self-interest *[documents 4 and 8b]*. Ball (1990: 16) summarises the application of the 'individualistic rational calculus' model of choice in education as being based upon the 'twin assumptions of egoism and utilitarianism' or, more generally, what Sen (1982: 16) has called the 'rational fools' and 'social morons' of 'purely economic man'.

Choice in education, as conceived by the reformers of the 1980s and 1990s, took a particular form. As Ball (1990: 10) argues, the emphasis was almost entirely upon giving 'the parent a limited role, confined to choice-making rather than involving participation in the life of the school. Here there is no room for voice, only for choice.' In doing so, as Miliband (1990: 14) suggests, the system devalues the parental role as producer of education, neglecting the vital contribution which they themselves make to a child's education.

Moreover, choice in education is most powerfully affected by what is available and accessible. Families in rural areas, served by only a single school for example, have little practical access to alternatives of any sort. In this regard, research evidence suggests that parents and prospective pupils draw on a range of non-educational rationales in reaching a choice of school. The Scottish research of Adler *et al.* (1989) concluded that proximity, security and achievement were the three factors most likely to be taken into account by choosers, with the first two seeming to take preference over the third. David *et al.* (1994: 21), who carried out a detailed investigation of the ways in which families, and especially mothers, understood and participated in the process of choosing a school, mirrored the Scottish findings in their identification of 'performance, proximity and pleasantness' as the criteria which most influenced parental choice of school.

Just as choice is mediated through a series of factors which lie outside the narrow definitions of educational performance, it is also likely to be shaped and influenced, as Glennerster (1996: 130) suggests, as much or more by the ability of the purchaser as it does on the quality of the producer. Issues of social class, race and gender all play a part in forming the unevenly distributed 'cultural capacities' which Gewirtz *et al.* (1995: 23) identify as the basis of three ideal types of choosers. They devise *privileged/skilled* choosers characterised, above all, by both the inclination and the capacity to choose, the *semi-skilled*, possessed of strong inclinations but limited capacity to engage with the market, and the *disconnected*, characterised by their disinclination to engage with the market.

Not only does choice involve more than educational considerations, and depend upon the characteristics of individual consumers, but it is also shaped by a series of other factors which casts doubt upon the 'neutrality' of choice and markets, as claimed by privatisation supporters. Evans and Vincent (1997: 113), in their account of choice within special education, suggest that far from being made up of the free-standing actors of neo-liberal formulation, the education market is shaped by a very particular ideation of its subjects. The incentive structures of the market lead schools to divide students into the 'desirable' and 'undesirable', a process which Glatter *et al.* (1997a: 126ff) conclude can generally be reduced to the attempt to attract 'more middle class parents'. Bowe *et al.* (1993: 53) make the same essential point slightly differently by phrasing it in explicitly commercial terms: 'The aim is not so much to ensure greater "value added" (as measured in terms of academic attainment) but to attract additional cultural capital into the school . . . hoping for higher yielding returns. Students bearing solid cultural capital look like good longer-term investments.'

Earlier parts of this chapter, dealing with GM schools and City Technology Colleges, have already suggested that where demand exceeds supply, choice shifts from consumer to producer. Rather than expand to accommodate the new demand, the evidence from education shows firmly that institutions prefer what Taylor-Gooby (1993: 115) calls 'the logic of status rather than growth', shaping that status through selection mechanisms, from money to academic achievement. Even where the situation is more fluid, however, the evidence cited above suggests, as Edwards and Whitty (1997: 40) conclude, that education markets operate in such a way that 'privileged producers and consumers will continue to search each other out in a progressive segmentation of the market'.

One of the central claims of the neo-liberals has been that individual choices, in a free market, combine to produce the best outcomes for all. As set out by Ranson (1990: 10), the application of this argument to the field of education suggests that 'although individuals only enter society and form associations to further their self-interest, nevertheless, the unintended consequence – guided by a hidden hand – is the general well-being of all in society'. Not only would the market enhance individual freedom, but it would also produce a spontaneous social order in which all would benefit, even if some would benefit more than others. The contention that the aggregate of individual choice in the market place amounts to an increase in the collective good is, however, difficult to maintain in the face of the evidence. In education, choices made by some actors appear clearly to have an impact upon the choices which remain for others. As Ball (1990: 13) suggests, 'In effect, the closure of an "unpopular" "local" school may result in considerable disadvantage for many families and a clear denial of preference . . . choices made by one set of parents [do not] actually leave the choices of others unaffected or undiminished', although 'this would seem to be the assumption upon which current legislation rests'. The Scottish research of Adler *et al.* (1989) found some 8–10 per cent of parents placing requests for their children to enter a school other than their local one, in both the primary and secondary sectors. The effects of these minority choices were cumulatively dramatic, leaving some local schools – the first choice of nine out of ten fellow parents – seriously under-enrolled and destabilised.

Miliband (1990: 9–11) addresses this issue at a higher level of generality. He quotes Ruth Jonathan (1989: 321) as concluding that 'only by ignoring the fact that individuals are socially located can we suppose that the welfare of each may be unproblematically aggregated to result in the welfare of all'. Yet, this is what, in essence, reliance upon the market produces. The individual decisions of parents produce an eventual class full of children in which their individual decisions interact in a way that has a significant impact upon the consequences that flow from the decisions made. Where these decisions are left to atomised individuals operating without reference to their collective interests, the result, Miliband (1990: 4) deduces, is a system in which 'the whole can be *less* than the sum of the parts, because of the way different elements interact'.

To summarise: choice in the education market of the 1980s and 1990s is a far more complex and ambiguous matter than the simple advantages claimed by the supporters of reform. The capacity to choose varies between individuals and the decisions made by some have consequences for others. As Hirsch (1977: 26) concludes: 'The choice offered by market opportunities are justly celebrated as liberating for the individual. Unfortunately, individual liberation does not make them liberating for all individuals together.' The choices made by individual actors are then combined with the choices and actions of producers, so as to shape the final market. Far from simply responding to the preferences of consumers, producers act deliberately to maximise their own advantage. In education this means encouraging the presence of students who appear to contribute to the aims of the institution, and its market position, while discouraging those who appear to act otherwise. The result is to produce a system characterised by competition rather than co-operation, and processes which result in losers as well as winners.

6.5 Privatisation, education and the individual

Two examples must suffice to illustrate this form of market operation upon individuals: open enrolment and school exclusion. Enhanced parental choice has been one of the most consistent themes of the New Right agenda in education. Measures to increase the power of parents in this way were included in every Education Act from 1980 onwards. Yet, ten years after the institution of 'open enrolment', evidence of the practical effects of choice in education is not encouraging. Late in 1996 the Audit Commission reported that one in five parents now failed to get their first choice of school, twice as many as previous official estimates, rising to almost a half in inner London schools. Open enrolment had resulted in one school in six being less than 75 per cent full – producing 900,000 empty places – while one in three had broken the government's restrictions on the number of pupils to be admitted. Market forces had thus failed to produce the closure of struggling schools, leaving local authorities with too little power to intervene in admissions and planning. In such circumstances, it is hardly surprising to find that appeals from parents in England against schools' admission decisions rose from 54,300 to 62,900 in 1995/96 and to 72,700 in 1996/97 (Department for Education 1998).

Concrete examples of what happens to those children who are not 'chosen' in the new system is provided by the London Borough of Bromley. Writing in 1993, Taylor-Gooby (1993: 115) recorded that, in the borough:

'Where twelve out of seventeen secondary schools are grant-maintained, 225 pupils were left without a secondary school place when admissions were announced in April 1992. Some students were later offered places in another borough and were faced with a twelve mile journey.'

By the summer of 1998, sixteen of the seventeen secondary schools in Bromley had become self-governing, grant-maintained establishments, able to select up to 15 per cent of their intake on the basis of academic ability. Competition, as driven by examination and other league tables, has resulted in Bromley schools recruiting able pupils from outside the Borough's own catchment area. The outcome has been, once again, that local children have to travel many miles further than their local school or, in the worst cases, outside the local authority altogether. Quoting the instance of a child travelling thirty miles each day to a school in Kent, *The Guardian* of 13 June 1998 reported that while Bromley has more than sufficient places for secondary school age children living within its own boundaries, 127 were unable to find a place in any Bromley school and were being obliged to travel outside the area for education. At the same time, Bromley problems were dwarfed by those in nearby Watford where 1,000 parents of children due to start secondary school in September 1998 were reported as not having been offered a place at any of the seven local schools, all of which had obtained grant-maintained status.

The second example, school exclusions, emerges from the claim that diversity and competition between schools would drive up standards for everyone. The contention was clearly put. Sexton (1987), for example – one of the most influential government advisers in this area – described the market as 'a built-in mechanism to raise standards and change forms and types of education in accordance with that market demand'.

Once again, the evidence which has emerged since implementation of the reforms has not been encouraging. Smith and Meier (1995) carried out a detailed empirical investigation of the school choice strategies in America, contrasting the claims made by the advocates of such strategies with their actual outcomes. Among their most significant finds are that 'embryonic school choice programs are associated with performance loss rather than gain'. In the British context, while examination results have improved since the 1988 reforms, these improvements began in the 1970s. Moreover, research suggests that only some 10 per cent of schools show significant, sustained improvement (see, for example, Gray 1996). League tables, in the meantime, may mask the extent to which any individual school is capable of 'adding value' to the abilities and capacities which pupils bring to its gate.

Dale (1997: 454), reviewing the literature concerning choice in the post-1988 system nearly ten years later, concluded that 'there is no evidence of any overall improvement in academic performance as a result of the introduction of school choice'. Bartlett et al. (1998: 7), reviewing the research of Whitty et al. (1998) in England, New Zealand and the USA conclude that: 'In none of the countries was there any evidence that increasing parental choice, either through introducing quasi-markets as in the UK or New Zealand, or through more participative programmes such as in some states of the USA, has had any impact at all on educational outcomes'.

For a significant proportion of the school population, in fact, the introduction of choice and competition in education has acted to worsen, rather than improve, the quality of their experience and its outcomes. The achievement in rate of examination passes is connected to a lowering in the number of pupils actually entered for public examinations. The proportion of students leaving school without any qualifications has grown over the same period as schools abandon the least able, targeting those marginal pupils who might, with extra investment, make a difference to league table results. Dale (1997: 463) summarises the findings of Gewirtz et al. (1995) in relation to students whom schools regard as market failures:

'Short termism, exemplified by exclusion policies: "passing the buck" on vulnerable students through the use of informal selection methods and associated self-exclusion; this is a phenomenon with a clear racial character: segregation policies, which operate both through streaming and response to Special Educational Needs: a narrowing of the scope of education, brought about in large part by new modes of performance monitoring: and a new hidden curriculum that places students as commodities.'

The impact of these processes upon those most directly affected has been a rapid escalation in the number of young people excluded from this form of public provision altogether. Figures provided by Hayden (1997), for example, show that recorded exclusions in all schools rose from 2,910 pupils in 1990/91 to 13,581 in 1995/96. Research reported by Hyams-Parish (1995) confirmed the view of schools as attributing this explosive rise firmly to market forces. Fully 87 per cent of schools identified 'increased competition between schools' as either the primary or secondary most significant explanation for the changing pattern of school exclusions.

The results of school exclusion do not fall at random upon the whole student population. The introduction of quasi-market forces into education marks out particular pupils as likely to detract from the image of individual schools through published league tables of attendance or examination success. Afro-Caribbean young men and pupils with special educational needs emerge regularly from survey results as far more vulnerable to exclusion than their numbers within the school population would warrant. Nor do these figures include those in the process of being statemented or those unofficially at home while the process is being negotiated. The integrationist policies of the 1981 Education Act are being rolled back by the competitive approach embodied within subsequent education reforms. Children with particular needs come to be perceived as a drain on school resources, and exclusion is one way in which that drain can be removed.

When a young person is excluded from school, direct costs (e.g. withdrawal of school meals) and indirect costs (e.g. on future employment opportunities) follow. At the end of the privatisation and marketisation processes which have been traced in this chapter lie the lives of individuals least able to bear the costs which are heaped onto them. It is difficult to be as sanguine as Bartlett *et al.* (1998: 1) who conclude their overview of marketisation and competition in social welfare with the view that, during this period, 'the principle of free and universal access, fundamental to the concept of the welfare state, was upheld'.

6.6 Summary

The account offered in this chapter demonstrates that the impact of privatisation upon education policy has been profound. Public assets have been transferred to private hands, while education itself has been transformed from a public to a private good. In the process, the fundamental basis of education provision has been altered. Citizenship, which suggests a concern for the well-being of others, has been replaced by consumerism, in which self-interest prevails.

For the marketeers, self-interest results in the best outcome not only for the individual but also for society as a whole. The conclusion suggested here is very different. Individual choices in education do not, in aggregate, deliver the benefits claimed. Rather, isolated actors, maximising their own best interests, combine incoherently to damage the prospects of others. The result is a system in which, across the school population as a whole, neither choice nor equity, efficiency or diversity can plausibly be said to have been enhanced.

Chapter 7

SOCIAL SERVICES

The social services, which form the focus of this chapter, differ in a number of key characteristics from the other social policy areas which are considered in this book. There are universal characteristics in health, education, social security and housing which mean that, at different times in their lives, almost all citizens will come into contact with these great services. Social services, by contrast, remain a minority field, with which most people, for the greater part of their lifetimes, will have almost no contact at all. When the personal social services are called upon, however, it is often to deal with an immediate crisis or a chronic difficulty. Over time, therefore, the scope of such services is substantial and the quality of services provided has a significant impact upon users.

As indicated in Chapter 1, the pattern of social service provision had always retained a substantial element of the 'mixed economy' of welfare, in which public services existed side-by-side with family, voluntary and charitable arrangements. At the same time, the level of state provision had grown substantially in the years immediately before and after the implementation of the Seebohm Report proposals in 1971. Lowe (1993: 271) suggests that, in the early period of Thatcher administration, the balance between annual expenditure between the different sectors stood at £400 million by charities, £3,800 million by the statutory social services and an estimated £24,000 million in services provided by informal care. The pattern, he suggested, 'confounded early postwar predictions' that non-public services would wither away under the welfare state.

This mixed pattern of provision struck two important chords with the incoming administration of 1979. On the one hand, it suggested that – unlike education or health, for example – the social services provided promising territory for increased private sector involvement and the promotion of a market in social care. On the other, it chimed with an even more fundamental Conservative instinct that the primary responsibility for care of this sort should lie, not with the state at all, but with families and charitable provision *[document 11a]*. The scene was thus set for policy efforts to increase the level of personal responsibility for obtaining help of a social services nature and for the creation of a more diverse pattern of provision through which that help might be obtained. The field thus offered fertile ground for the general policy thrust which Giddens (1998: 27) expresses as the 'paradoxical mix of economic libertarianism and moral traditionalism' of the Thatcher administrations. In the account which follows, two essential strategies are explored – the development of charging policies (particularly in relation to the social care of older people, by far the largest group to be affected by the changes) and the evolution of a contract culture in the provision of personal social services.

7.1 Charging

As other chapters have demonstrated, one of the primary means through which the privatisers and free-market sponsors of the New Right sought to increase personal responsibility during the 1980s was by making the price of services more explicit and by charging direct users a greater proportion of the costs of service provision. During the post-1979 period, two new pressures were applied to extend charging in the social services into new areas and to fresh dimensions. On the one hand, as Kendall *et al.* (1997: 186) suggest, the long-standing radical right argument that 'the market is generally superior to the ballot box as a means of registered consumer preference' (Lees 1965: 76) came to be applied with vigour to the social services arena. From this perspective, the rationing which has always been a part of such provision is simply more honestly and transparently organised through the price mechanism than the arbitrary and secret procedures of public bureaucrats. On the other, and even more significantly, the shift of responsibility for the care of older people from the health to the social services (as explored further in Chapter 8) represented a paradigm alteration in responsibility from free to means-tested services. Such a shift, of course, in the terms of this book, represents a reallocation of responsibilities, both within the state and from the state to the individual. 'Cost-shunting', as it is known, is a phenomenon in which one service attempts to shed its financial responsibility by transferring it elsewhere. In the process, substantial energies become caught up in 'boundary wars', in which organisations attempt to fend off such attempts. The boundary between health and social care remains the most significant example in community care, but by no means the only one. Clapham *et al.* (1994: 2), for example, trace the 'hotly disputed' boundary which can arise between social services and housing authorities, in cases where the distinction between 'care costs' (which should fall to social services) and 'housing management costs (which should fall to the housing authority) are difficult to separate or define. In such circumstances, considerable energy can be deflected from considering the best interests of individuals and into the self-protection of agency budgets. In whatever ways state agencies may attempt to shunt costs between one another, the individual is very likely to end up paying more. The boundary between public and private responsibility will have been shifted to place a greater burden upon the latter.

Charging and residential care

The essential facts of the changing arrangement for funding long-term care are set out by Wistow (1997). In his phrase, the emerging market in private and residential care during the 1980s, funded by social security payments, represented a 'silent social revolution' in the care of older people. Hospital beds for older patients fell from 55,600 in 1976 to 37,500 in 1994, while mental health beds for older people also fell from 26,500 to 18,200 between 1988 and 1996 (House of Commons Health Committee, 1995). At the same time, average length of stay fell by one-third, while throughput increased by over 80 per cent and day case surgery grew by more than 200 per cent (DoH 1994). Proportionately, older people were affected to the greatest extent by these changes.

At the same time, a four-fold increase (to 358,000) took place in the number of residential and nursing home places provided by the independent sectors. Wistow (1997: 107) shows how this growth led, in just over twenty years, to a reversal in the respective roles of the public and independent sectors as care providers for older people: 'in the 1970s, 69% of all long-term care in institutional settings for older, physically disabled and chronically ill people was provided within NHS or local government facilities. Yet, by 1994, those proportions had switched to 24% and 76% respectively' (Laing and Buisson 1995).

The funding for this major change came through the social security budget which now came, in effect, to provide a massive subsidy to the health service, by picking up the costs for those who had previously been looked after in hospital. At the same time, cash-starved local authorities added to these pressures by taking advantage of social security regulations to buy themselves out of direct responsibility for older people. The number of residents supported by the DHSS rose from 16,000 to 281,000 between 1982 and 1993 and the cost of supporting them rose from £39 million to £2,575 million over the same period (House of Commons Health Committee 1995). In terms of charging, of course, this change represents the scale of shift from full state responsibility to the conditional responsibility of means-testing. Only 5 per cent of the 194,000 nursing home residents in 1994 were funded by the NHS (Laing and Buisson 1995). All the others were subjected to means-testing. For those who were entitled to assistance from the DHSS, however, as Lunt *et al.* (1996: 372) suggest, payment 'served as a voucher system, which was directly under the control of users who qualified for the allowance'. In that sense, the new system exhibited powerful market characteristics, placing the power of purchase in the hands of individuals and generating a supply to match the new demand. Becker (1997: 124) illustrates the scale of this market development when noting that between 1982 and 1992 the number of residents in private homes increased by almost 260 per cent, while the numbers in local authority homes fell by 32 per cent. 'By 1995', as he suggests, 'the private sector accounted for more than three-quarters of all places in residential care homes . . . [it] had grown from a relatively small-scale provider of residential and nursing home care, to become the market leader'.

From a political perspective, the threat of means-testing became especially problematic as it clashed with the promotion of home ownership, another key policy priority. More than half of those aged over 60 are now owner-occupiers, and the average value of a house is some £60,000. The impact of means-testing upon such assets were, as Wistow (1997: 109) suggests, 'to penalise savings [and] discourages self reliance and provides incentives for elderly people to divest themselves of their assets in order to avoid liability for such payments'. Becker (1997: 140) describes the process as one of 'institutional impoverishment' of older people in which, 'as their frailty progressed and their savings declined, they were transformed from independent citizens in the community, to financially independent users of residential care services, to the dependent poor in institutions'. The result, in the terms used by the Joseph Rowntree Foundation *Inquiry into Meeting the Costs of Continuing Care* (JRF 1996), has been to place the assets of a minority of older people at 'catastrophic risk' through means-testing, while, for the majority, engendering a sense of a 'broken contract' with the State in which their contributions have been either disregarded – in terms of payment of tax and national insurance – or, in terms of savings, positively used against them.

Charging and the Community Care Act 1990

During the 1980s, the changes outlined above proceeded relatively piece-meal and without overall direction. The policy consequences were drawn together in the 1990 NHS and Community Care Act. Henwood *et al.* (1996: 40) set out the sequence of events leading up to the Act. A series of critical reports concerning the consequences of the changing boundary between health and social care – what Deakin (1996: 27) refers to as 'two markets grinding against each other' – and the quality of services to be found in the community sector, led to the commissioning of a review of these issues from Sir Roy Griffiths, one of the Government's favourite trouble-shooters. He reported in 1988, but his preferred solution – that local authorities should be given lead responsibility for care in the community, including a transfer of funding from the DHSS – was received only reluctantly by Ministers. Fifteen months went by before, as Wistow and Henwood (1991) suggest, the Griffiths model was accepted by Government 'as the "least bad option", only after an extensive search for an alternative model'. By then, as Rhodes (1992: 67) points out, a further string in the privatising armoury of the government had contributed to a lessening of the power of local government to stand in the way of central determination. In London, for example, the abolition of the Greater London Council, and its replacement by 'a range of bodies including central departments, quangos, private companies, joint bodies, joint committees, district councils/London boroughs' had produced a situation in which 'only 33 per cent of the expenditure on local services in London is by the directly elected London boroughs'. The removal of decision making from the public to the private sphere was thus part of the context in which the privatisation of services previously delivered by local councils could take place.

In terms of privatisation, the economic changes which Griffiths produced involved a further move away from state responsibility. Lunt *et al.* (1996: 372) point out that the DHSS funding of residential care places was demand-led rather than cash-limited. Under the new arrangements, 'so far as the central government is concerned, the budget for community care is now cash limited, in the sense that its commitment is limited by the grants it chooses to transfer to local authorities'. The implications of cash-limiting, in terms of charges for local authority domiciliary services, are discussed in more detail below. The impact upon charges for residential care were researched by Laing (1998: 1), who concluded that 'frequent disparities' existed 'between the fees that state agencies are willing to pay and the full, reasonable cost of long-term care'. In his estimate, £80 million each year is currently spent on '"top-ups" to bridge the visible disparities between care home fees and what state agencies are willing to pay'. The bulk of this sum is found by residents' families, thus adding further to the transfer of responsibility from services previously provided free of charge to those now imposed upon individuals. While market theory might have suggested that residential fees would have been driven lower, in order to balance supply with demand, Laing (1998: 6) concludes that for-profit providers have reacted by withdrawing totally from activity in the field. Others, such as Lapsley and Llewellyn (1998: 147), suggest that the funding differentials which have opened up between those who depend upon the state and those who can pay for themselves is then reflected in differential standards of care – with best rooms, for example, reserved for self-funders – 'the quality of care for LA funded clients may then be compromised and class divisions may be perpetuated in such homes'.

The NHS and Community Care Act formalised the separation of health service and community responsibilities. It led to an acceleration of the withdrawal of hospital services for the continuing care of older people. The change proved to be continuingly controversial. Henwood *et al.* (1996: 46), in their research of the practice in five different localities, conclude that the public became more aware of their rights to free NHS care as the prospects of receiving that care diminished. Providers in all five places reported 'pressure from relatives to keep patients in NHS care'. Thus, one of the essential purposes of privatisation in the social policy area came under increasing scrutiny and political pressure. The NHS and Community Care Act received the Royal Assent on 29 June 1990. It did not come fully into operation until April 1993. Less than two years later, in 1995, the Department of Health published new guidelines intended, according to Henwood *et al.* (1996: 47), to 'halt the withdrawal of the NHS from continuing care . . . [thus] moving that line back towards the NHS'.

7.2 Social services and the contract culture

The transfer of responsibilities and budgets to local authorities under the 1990 Act was organised, in the first instance, on the basis of a ring-fenced Special Transitional Grant (STG), designed to protect expenditure in this new area from the competing claims of other local authority services. That grant, however, was subject to particular conditions, said by some commentators to be the price which Mrs Thatcher demanded for agreeing to increasing the responsibilities of the hated local authorities. No more than 15 per cent of the STG was to be spent on in-house services. The remainder was to be devoted to purchasing from the private, independent and voluntary sectors. The result was to distinguish the purchase of personal social services from the 'internal' market arrangements of, for example, the health service reforms. As Mannion and Smith (1998: 112) suggest, 'the principal features of community care which distinguish it from these other publicly-funded quasi-markets is that it is an *external* market, in which providers are drawn predominantly from the independent sector, and that many of the providers are likely to be profit-seeking' (original emphasis).

In Becker's (1997: 122) description, the new arrangement exhibited

> 'the essential ingredients of New Right thinking, namely that the direct involvement of the state in welfare matters should be limited to support a vibrant pluralist economy of care, combining the best of private enterprise with voluntary and charitable giving, subject to the discipline and rigour of a free market, within the framework of the law. This was coupled with the policy imperative to reduce public expenditure on social programmes, particularly on cash and care.'

The claims which accompanied the introduction of community care were thus the familiar ones: that the greater introduction of market principles into the purchase and provision of social services would bring benefits of independence, choice, quality and economy, to be achieved by generating competition – 'the founding principle' of the new arrangements according to Charlesworth et al. (1996: 70) – among suppliers and the provision of freedom to consumers of services to pursue their own interests in the market place.

Purchasing services

In the years since community care was implemented, a considerable body of evidence has grown up which throws light upon the essential claims of those responsible for its introduction. A number of the questions raised by this evidence replicates the concerns highlighted through investigation of similar processes in other social policy areas. The role of purchaser in community care services, for example, faces the same ambiguities which arise in the case of GP fundholders. The self-interested and skilful consumer, upon whom so much market theory depends, stands at one remove from the pursuit of community care services. The final user is only a 'proxy customer' (Charlesworth et al. 1996:

77) of services which are purchased, in fact, by an agent, the community care manager. This device not only weakens one of the most important theoretical pillars of marketisation but relies upon a contradiction within it. In the view taken by public choice theory, as Chapter 2 explained more fully, employees of the welfare state emerged as discredited figures, cloaking the pursuit of their own interests under spurious claims to professionalism and a public service ethos. The break-up of public monopolies and the enfranchisement of consumers was the cure for this inherently anti-user outcome. In the quasi-markets of community care, however, as Lewis *et al.* (1996: 3) suggest, the rejected notions of professionalism have to be 'dusted off' as the system can only work if the purchasing agents – the community care managers – can be assumed to be motivated by 'the wish to maximise the welfare of users'. Bartlett *et al.* (1998: 4) put this dilemma most positively when they suggest that, 'Quasi-markets may operate best where they are structured to capture the positive effect of both private and altruistic motivations of welfare service providers.' The achievability of such a structure, however, is at least open to question.

In practice, the assumption that the anti-user villains of state welfare would be transformed into the user-champions of the market place became subject to a series of conflicting pressures which revealed some basic dilemmas planted at the heart of the community care legislation. The Griffiths Report and subsequent pronouncements by government laid great stress upon the *needs-led* character of the new service. Unlike the previous system, which – as the marketeers argued – had been dominated by state interests, the new approach would put the consumer first. The process would begin with an assessment of the needs of any individual requiring care in the community, and that statement of need would then drive the process forward. 'Care managers', as they were now to be known, would be responsible for constructing flexible packages of services, drawn largely from the responsive non-state sector and tailored to meet these individual needs. The bad old days, in which individuals were shoe-horned into a limited number of services, directly provided by the local authorities and designed to suit their own vested interests, were to be over.

On implementation, the needs-led approach soon met the constraints of a cash-limited service. The Association of Directors of Social Services had, from the outset, complained that the cash allocation from central government for the new community care services was less than half of the sum required to discharge the new responsibilities. These predictions were quickly borne out once the system came into operation. Becker (1997: 135–6) describes the outcome as exposing the 'deceit in community care implementation'. Far from being needs-led, the system fell back rapidly, in Becker's words, upon 'the use of assessment, prioritizing and eligibility criteria . . . to regulate and ration access to expensive forms of care, both residential, nursing and domiciliary, for users and carers'.

Lewis *et al.* (1996), drawing on research evidence from a series of local authority areas, reach a number of conclusions which illustrate Becker's contentions in practice and add a new layer of complexity to them. In these findings, even those authorities most enthusiastic for the new arrangements, and committed

109

to the principles upon which they had been promoted, found themselves struggling with difficulties of implementation. One of the central difficulties which this study identifies is, again, familiar from other quasi-market systems – that of inadequate or asymmetric information. At a whole-system level such deficiencies included the fact that 'provider systems are not geared to producing information about costs in the manner required by purchasers' (Lewis *et al.* 1996: 10). Moreover, purchasers are often not in a position to know when costs are being artificially inflated or misallocated by providers, a problem which, as discussed more fully below, grows the more systems attempt to provide differentiated rather than bulk services. As Ranade (1998: 12) suggests in a similar context, 'the regulated know more about their businesses than the regulators and are usually in a good position to outwit them'. At an individual level, information deficits produce what Lewis *et al.* (1996: 10) refer to as 'the kinds of invoicing problems commonly referred to in the literature (e.g. Le Grand 1993), with examples of billing for dead clients and for clients who have not received service, and the purchase orders necessary for the tracking of purchasing commitments not being routinely filed or even properly numbered'. The result of these difficulties has been a 'vast increase in bureaucracy, as more forms feed burgeoning information and information technology systems' (Lewis *et al.* 1996: 17). 'Transaction costs' as they are known, thus eat away at two of the major claims for market systems – those of economy and efficiency.

Mannion and Smith (1998: 114) develop this argument in two important ways. Firstly, they point to the considerable distance which, in practice, separates the social care manager from the rational economic actors of neo-liberal theory. Operating in a market which the authors describe as 'about as complex a market as can be envisaged', care managers are adversely affected not only by asymmetry of information (knowing less about services than service providers), but also 'bounded rationality', that is to say, by the difficulties of processing the amount of information necessary to make rational choices, even if that information were to be available. The effect of these circumstances, Mannion and Smith suggest, is to reinforce the tendency of care managers to be 'risk averse'. Working in a context where the impact of market failure – such as the closure of a private residential home – would be very significant for service users, care managers are likely to weigh up the impact which their decisions make upon these wider environmental risks. Their responses, tempered by asymmetry and bounded rationality, result in what Bartlett *et al.* (1998: 8) summarise as a tendency 'to restrict the provision of care to a fortunate privileged few, since fixed budget constraints prohibited the purchase of large quantities of high quality services'. As a later section of this chapter demonstrates, 'restriction' of services in this way is synonymous with 'rationing'. Here, a more general point needs to be drawn out which Roberts *et al.* (1998: 286) make when they identify rationing within the quasi-market as a means of obfuscating state responsibility for adequate funding of necessary services. In their conclusion, the reduced number of individuals receiving community care services 'links the whole initiative back to the central philosophy of rolling back the state, supporting [the] view that quasi-markets potentially provide a buffer for central authorities, deflecting responsibility from governments'. The privatisation of responsibility has been identified as a consistent theme in the social policy areas considered in this book. Community care is no exception.

Providing services

If purchasers found difficulties in the new market place, the pattern of suppliers anticipated in the 1990 Act also failed to meet the ambitions which had been set out for them. Local authorities, faced with having to spend at least 85 per cent of their transitional grant in the non-state sector, were obliged to externalise in-house services, not only to preserve the employment of those engaged in them, but also to make up for the absence of sufficient independent providers through whom services at the 85 per cent level might be obtained. In some instances this has amounted, according to Roberts *et al.* (1998: 277), to a failure not simply to create a real market, but even to 'ensure that the markets were at least contestable'. Even where providers were available, the advantages of responsiveness, economy and quality claimed for them, were not always readily apparent. Lewis *et al.* (1996: 13), for example, quote from one of the local authorities included in their research who 'reported that a 1994 market mapping exercise revealed that 50 per cent of the domiciliary care agencies identified in 1992 no longer existed'. Even when providers are available, the advantages of responsiveness and individually tailored packages of care have not always been forthcoming. During the 1980s, the rapid growth of private residential care for older people had already provided evidence that profit, rather than variety or value, drove the market. Consumers whose needs fell outside the narrow confines of the balance sheet were faced more by intensifying neglect than an enhanced choice of services (Langan 1990). The failure of the market to respond to the needs of older black and minority ethnic communities, for example, well illustrated the way in which the requirements of a dominant – in this case, white – consumer group drive out the needs of less powerful actors in the market place (see, for example, National Council for Voluntary Organisations 1989). By the end of the decade, private residential homes were part of the portfolio of such as Ladbroke plc and the brewers Vaux and Boddingtons, organisations whose track-record of interest in social welfare was difficult to establish and by whom the care of older people was bought and sold as any other commodity on the stock exchange (Drakeford 1993).

The problems of providing for particular needs within a market system have not disappeared with the introduction of community care. Means and Langan (1996: 258), for example, report on the development of services for older people with dementia under the new arrangements. They conclude that such individuals are 'unattractive to service providers'. That unattractiveness is overcome, essentially, only by a financial compensation sufficient to outweigh the 'difficulties and challenges generated by this client group' (p. 258). In these circumstances, market actors operate to protect or promote their own financial interests. Providers of care use the power which shortage of supply generates to raise prices. Because the exercise of financial responsibilities by older people with dementia is complex and problematic, suppliers emerged, in the Means and Langan study, as 'cream-skimming' purchasers – preferring those local authorities most prepared to meet the full costs themselves. Local authorities, in turn, had a clear interest in either recovering such costs from individuals concerned or minimising the costs generated in other ways. Thus researchers concluded that, at some time, practice in all the local authorities surveyed was 'primarily concerned with the need to establish effective revenue collection strategies . . . rather than from a desire to protect vulnerable elderly people and to act as advocates on their behalf'. Where cost recovery was too problematic, an alternative strategy simply avoided recognition of the particular needs of elderly people with dementia, so that 'they were processed relatively cheaply in terms of financial assessment and fee collection along with the rest of the "elderly"'.

7.3 Outcomes in the contract culture

Block contracts or spot purchase?

Information difficulties, the pressures of finance and the state of the market, push even those authorities reluctant to do so in the direction of block contracts and 'set-list' services. Common and Flynn (1992), in an early investigation of the separation of purchaser and provider roles within local authorities, concluded that the substitution of a monopoly private provider for a monopoly public service was widespread. One of Lewis et al.'s respondents (1996: 15) suggested that block contracts were preferred because they provided the advantages of lower unit costs, reduced transaction costs and as a result 'of the problems of monitoring quality in respect of numerous spot contracts and because independent providers were refusing to provide small numbers of hours of service'. Even where care managers were provided with more-than-usual freedom to make spot purchases in order to meet individual needs, this study found that they were 'more likely to draw off the centrally commissioned menu of services first because it is administratively easier'. Such findings stand in stark contrast to the recommendations of studies which attempt to develop ideas for user-centred approaches. Clapham et al. (1994: 3), for example, suggest that systems which aim to meet individual needs with more precision should adopt spot purchasing 'as the norm'. The reality appears to be that, as community care has become established, 'off-the shelf' rather than bespoke services are, in fact, the norm for most service users in all authorities (see, for example, Baldock and Ungerson 1994 and Hoyes et al. 1994). It is within that context that Becker (1997: 139) quotes the Audit Commission's (1996) description of the process of assessment and prioritising care needs by local authority care managers as bearing 'a striking resemblance to the process of "considered decision making" adopted by social fund officers with regards to care needs'.

The relative absence of power among purchasers stands in contrast to the anticipated outcomes of those marketisation theories upon which the transformation of services into purchaser and provider units was based. Nor are these findings confined to circumstances where providers are at a premium. Smith (1996: 113) reports the experience of the United States, where 'many states and localities rely entirely on private agencies funded by contracts to deliver important public services, including child protection, home care and residential care for the mentally ill'. In practice, however, this situation does not arise from an active market, made up of a plethora of competing suppliers. Rather, a series of serious disincentives to the disruption of existing relationships means that contracts are usually renewed with existing suppliers, that genuine competition is rare and that efficiency gains are often elusive. Among the disincentives are the loss of trust which competitive tendering produces, the disruption which this causes in other relationships in which different parties are engaged, as well as the financial costs which can dissuade new entrants from entering the competitive process. Moreover, as Smith (1996: 117) suggests, contracts are rarely switched to new agencies because this would 'at the very least require the purchasing agency to justify its decision under the glare of public scrutiny. Terminating contracts can be very difficult because of the elusiveness of outcome measures.' In the United Kingdom, Deakin (1996: 36), reporting the results of a study of contracts and the public sector in social care, concludes that 'cartels are already forming; and there is much lazy use of block contracts'.

Choice and responsiveness

Block contracts and unchanging contractors, of course, deny one of the main claims which the marketisation of social services was meant to bring about – choice and responsiveness in a plural market of suppliers and purchasers. They also undermine claims in relation to what Lewis et al. (1996: 17) term the 'acknowledged Achilles heel of markets', the question of quality. Henwood et al. (1996: 49) suggest that this problem, particularly, is compounded by the organisation of community care services through proxy purchase arrangements. Older people face the realistic fear that declining health and other capacities will lead to the need for a greater level of assistance in the future, if they are to be enabled to continue living in the community. That knowledge creates a hesitation in appearing demanding or persistent in relation to present need, in case a reputation for 'troublemaking' may prejudice future provision. Even where such anxiety might be ill-founded, its understandable presence prevents the wholehearted pursuit of immediate self-interest through which the benefits of market systems are said to be derived.

Deakin (1996: 29) reports the views of voluntary and for-profit providers of social care within the British social services market. In response to an attitude questionnaire, no set of purchasers or providers agreed that 'quality of service usually improves as a result of contracts'. Within public sector purchasers, 32 per cent agreed, while 35 per cent disagreed with the proposition. Voluntary sector providers were even less impressed, with only 15 per cent in agreement with the proposition that contracts usually improved quality, while 36 per cent disagreed. Even for-profit providers could not muster a majority in favour. Here 29 per cent both agreed and disagreed with the statement.

If such levels of scepticism exist among key players in relation to the benefits of markets in social care, Deakin's (1996: 34) account attempts to identify those whose interests have been served by the changes. In his conclusion, for-profit organisations emerge as more optimistic about the benefits of the new system than voluntary sector bodies, while, in terms of the purchasers of care, 'there is little doubt about who the gainers are: it has been the senior managers whose role has expanded and who stand to gain both materially and professionally as a result'. The co-option of senior managerial staff to the privatisation project is a general theme in both economic and social policy areas. Bartlett *et al.* (1998: 2), for example, conclude that 'in nearly all areas, the reforms were at first fiercely resisted by the professional cadres in the different sectors, only to be welcomed eventually by some in those same groups as a result of the increased levels of managerial autonomy and discretion that they introduced'. By contrast, Deakin's view of users – to whom this chapter now turns – was that those 'who were meant to be the chief beneficiaries of the reforms have not been participants to any significant extent in the dialogue about the future direction of policy'.

Rationing and the individual

Whatever the difficulties faced within the internal market, one theme seems clear and consistent: that new arrangements and increasing financial constraint have combined to produce more explicit rationing of community-based services and a greater use of charging for those services when they are made available.

The explicit case for rationing – or targeting, to use the term preferred by its supporters – is made by Davies (1997: 340) when he suggests that, prior to the 1990 Act, community services were too thinly spread, providing assistance with tasks which recipients 'claimed to be able to undertake without difficulty'. A concentration of resources upon those most in need is thus justified on the basis that it helps those who require it most, without damaging others too severely. For those on the receiving end of cuts, however, the picture does not appear so sanguine. According to research carried out by the Personal Social Services Research Unit at the University of Manchester, eligibility criteria for services differ widely in form, context, reliability and quality from one part of the country to another. As a result, outcomes are uncertain at best, and arbitrary at worst. Davies' contention that criteria are driven by the search for more effective patterns of spending appears at odds with the findings of others (such as Wright 1997) who emphasise that tightening eligibility is driven by the search to control spending through reducing the number of people entitled to receive services.

The 1983 Health and Social Services and Social Security Adjudications Act (HSSSSAA) provides local authorities with discretionary powers to charge for domiciliary care services, provided the charges are 'reasonable' and reviewable in the light of changing circumstances. The services covered include home care, day care, meals-on-wheels and aids and adaptations. While local authorities are not obliged to charge, the Conservative government assumed that charges for domiciliary services would be levied in setting the level of annual central government grant which councils receive. Specifically, government set a level of 9 per cent of the costs of non-residential adult services to be recovered through charges in this way. The Local Government Anti-Poverty Unit (1995: 1) pinpoints the essential dilemma which this produces for social services authorities: 'to raise revenue from charges to ensure that service levels are maintained whilst not impoverishing individual users. These two objectives are incompatible. All that local authorities can do is trade one off against the other.'

Becker (1997: 143–4) shows how the 1990 Act has marked a watershed in the practical approach of local authorities to charging for services provided in the home. During the 1980s, he argues, councils generally attempted to keep down charges as much as possible. In the 1990s, however, 'the government has actively encouraged the use of charges wherever possible for community care services'. Based on the assumption that cost recovery at the 9 per cent level would be achieved, central grant to local authorities was reduced by £260 million in 1995/96, regardless of the actual level of any income received by authorities nationally or locally. In practice this assumption did not reflect the circumstances of most authorities. In two-thirds of cases councils reported failure to raise this level of revenue through charges both because of the cost of collection and, as Becker notes, 'user resistance to paying'. The impact of the funding regime was to advantage those areas where users were most likely to be able to pay and, through short-falls in central funding for those unable to meet the 9 per cent target, to penalise local authorities whose residents needed help the most. Becker reports, for example, that Buckingham was able to raise 18.4 per cent of its social services spending in charges, while the London Borough of Waltham Forest raised just 1.4 per cent in the same way.

One of the recurring themes of this book has been the way in which marketisation, and the privatisation of responsibilities hitherto accepted by the public sphere, add to the disadvantage of those who already carry the heaviest burden. Charges for domiciliary services in social work form part of this same pattern. Nor are such pressures always mitigated by the way in which local authorities discharge their often-reluctant decision to raise revenue. Baldwin and Lunt (1996: 1), in their review of council charging policies, found widespread concern among authorities 'about the possible effects of charging users, including: reduced use of services; increased financial hardship; poorer quality of life; bad effects on user-professional relationships'. Yet, the same authors discovered practice which added to, rather than mitigated these effects. Charging policies were variable, complex and driven by 'irresistible' financial imperatives. Most authorities operated a minimum charge for all users, based on a mixture of flat-rate charges and means-testing. The result was that those receiving Income Support were left with an income below that very basic level.

Within this complex and increasing recourse to charging, the same variability which characterised eligibility criteria was also repeated. Kempson (1997: 3), for example, found that the cost of a single item, such as meals-on-wheels, varied from £10.50 a week in the most expensive part of the country to £3.10 in the cheapest. Moreover, while most of the areas identified as low cost for meals-on-wheels made no charge for home care services, such charges were levied in all the high-cost areas. The Baldwin and Lunt (1996: 4) study tested the operation of council policies against the basic criteria set out in the 1983 HSSSSA Act, concluding that, 'the study found that policies operating in all six areas fell short of reasonableness at a great many levels'.

The combined result of these developments, as Becker (1997: 145) suggests, has been 'to distort demand, deterring poor people who need home care from applying for it and deflecting services to more wealthy elderly people who need them less'. The charity Scope has reported that almost one in five disabled people had to turn down some care from social services because they could not afford to meet the charges. In common with the findings of earlier chapters, therefore, charging policies in the social services have been found to play their part in the privatisation of social policy. As the state has pulled back from supporting those who had previously been able to rely upon its assistance, so the boundary between public and private has been redrawn, leaving such individuals to make their own arrangements. The invigorating release of individual effort, initiative and enterprise which the New Right identified as most likely to follow such a policy has turned out to be wanting. People whose circumstances were already strained and constrained have found yet further limitation rather than liberation to be the outcome.

As in all other areas of social policy considered in this book, the 1979–97 Conservative administrations maintained an active record of policy making in relation to social services right up to the General Election of May 1997. In November 1994, for example, the Secretary of State for Health and Social Services, Virginia Bottomley, announced plans which would allow direct payments to be made from social services to disabled people, in order to allow them directly to purchase their own care services, rather than through community care arrangements. The necessary legislation completed its parliamentary stages in July 1996. The scheme was publicised as resolving the difficulties of choice and independence which had emerged in social care quasi-markets. In practice, as Becker (1997: 151) demonstrates, it was an independence heavily hedged with caveats:

> 'there will be no automatic entitlement to payments . . . there is no compulsion – which, in effect will mean that there will be wide geographical variations, as with charging policies. Moreover, while the user is to decide what to purchase, SSDs must agree on how the money will be spent and users must show that their choice is as cost-effective as the package that could be provided or arranged by social services.'

Early in 1997, continuing anxieties about the funding of the long-term care of an increasing population of older people produced a set of proposals based around the encouragement of private insurance cover for care, on a public/private partnership model developed in parts of America. Evidence for the success of such a model was far from straightforward. Burchardt and Hills (1997: 4), for example, in their general survey of the financial implications of replacing state provision through private insurance arrangements, concluded that long-term care was 'a most unsuitable risk to be covered privately except for a small, relatively wealthy, healthy group (mostly men)'. Of all the potential areas for insurance cover, this presented the greatest difficulties, with uncertainties around future care needs and costs making alternative policies 'virtually impossible to assess, for both consumers and providers'.

In the dying days of the 1997 Conservative Government, a social services White Paper *Achievement and Challenge* was published on 12 March *[document 11a]*. It suggested reviewing the direct payments scheme to younger disabled people and extending it to cover other categories of need. The powers of local authorities to provide direct residential care services for older people were to be confined only to those circumstances where it could be demonstrated that such needs could not be met in the independent sector. A similar determination to encourage and facilitate a further increase in the independent sector provision of non-residential care was also included. The notion that neo-liberal radicalism had departed from Conservative administration turns out not to bear scrutiny. The theme of private good and public bad continued to characterise the administration's approach to the social services until its demise, with active plans in preparation for a continuation of the privatisation project should the electorate have given its approval.

7.4 Summary

The tradition of voluntary effort in the social services meant it provided some of the more promising ground for shifting the boundary between public and private provision within the field of social welfare. The belief that care was a primary responsibility of families themselves was a long-standing part of the Conservative tradition upon which the more radical methods of neo-liberalism were able to build. The themes of private insurance, cost-transference and marketisation which have been explored in this chapter have already been found in different ways among the other services discussed in Part Two of this book. The effect has been to residualise even further the public provision of social services, with 'reserved for the poor' hung ever more firmly above the door of local authority social services offices. This tightening of the net leaves outside it a growing group of those left to provide for themselves. Private sector services, bought from their private pockets, are to be their solution. As this chapter has demonstrated, however, where that prescription cannot be applied, the resulting difficulties are ones which the state has become less and less willing to address.

Chapter 8

HEALTH

The Bill which created the National Health Service received the Royal Assent in November 1946. It formed the centre piece of the great reforming programme of the post-war Labour administration and one of the main pillars of the new Welfare State.

This chapter returns to the founding principles of public welfare, as explored in Chapter 1 and exemplified in the NHS. It sets out the problems identified by those who favoured a greater private presence, the solutions which such proponents proposed and the beneficial outcomes which were claimed, should such prescriptions be applied. It will then go on to investigate and assess these claims against the actual policy regimes applied to the National Health Service since 1979.

8.1 Founding principles

Any attempt to consider the changes introduced to the National Health Service during the 1980s and 1990s needs to begin with an understanding of the principles upon which the service was originally founded. Powell (1996: 27ff) provides a useful discussion of the basis of the 1946 National Health Service, drawing on the testimony of its first Minister, Aneurin Bevan. The essential principles which emerge may be summarised as:

- *Equality of access* The service was to be open to all on the simple basis of citizenship or residence. In Bevan's words, the 'resources of medical skill and apparatus of healing shall be . . . made available to rich and poor alike' (Bevan 1978: 99–100). The disqualifying criteria which were characteristic of means-tested or insurance-based services – in which lack of money or threshold criteria often resulted in care being denied at the point when it was most needed – were to be abandoned. As Cooper and Culyer (1971: 3) suggest: 'The link between contribution and benefit, fundamental to twentieth century British social policy, was abandoned.'
- *Equity in treatment* Not only was the service to be made available to all, but all would be treated in the same way within it. The sole test by which treatment was to be applied was medical need, or to quote Bevan (1978: 103)

118

again, 'the essence of a satisfactory health service is that the rich and the poor are treated alike, that poverty is not a disability and that wealth is not advantaged'. Equity in treatment embodied a concern with equality of outcome, as well as access. Not only was the health service to be equally open to all, but it was to provide results on the same basis.

- *Comprehensive in provision*   The health service was to be distinguished from the piecemeal pattern of private provision which it replaced by its comprehensive character. It was thorough-going, not only in being available to all citizens, but by providing the full range of services which illness or disease might require.
- *Free at the point of use*   The single most distinctive feature of the new health service was to be the elimination of cash transactions at the point of medical need. Collective services were to be collectively financed, through the tax system. Neither patient nor doctor was to have the spectre of finance intruding upon a decision to seek medical help or the decision as to which forms of help should be provided. As Powell (1996: 29) suggests, it was 'the combination of the free and universal objectives that were the hallmark of the NHS'.

The NHS thus unambiguously asserted the advantages of public over private forms of provision. In Bevan's (1978: 109) words: 'A free health service is a triumphant example of the superiority of collective action and public initiative applied to a segment of society where commercial principles are seen at their worst.' On the grounds of economy and ethics, public service was to be preferred to the market *[document 2]*.

8.2 The privatiser's lament

From the perspective of those who believed that the 1946 settlement represented a basic miscalculation between the relative merits of public and private provision, the problems which faced the Health Service were not so much the accidental or unforeseeable by-product of a heroic experiment, as inevitable and intrinsic to the whole venture *[document 3]*. The arguments which emerged form part of that general re-evaluation of public welfare which was traced in Chapter 2. The specific problems in relation to health, from this perspective, included:

- *The denial of essential freedom.* In a system weighted heavily in favour of collective provision, the individual is constrained. Choice and diversity suffer as the system places barriers in the path of, and heaps costs upon, those who seek to depart from it. In the process the total stock of freedom is diminished.
- *The absence of financial discipline at the point of service delivery.* Free at the point of use, in this argument, also means an irresponsible freedom from accountability for the real costs which any service implies. Where neither producers nor consumers of health services bear the consequences of their decisions there are, as Maynard (1995: 71) suggests, 'few incentives to economise and

use resources efficiently'. Moreover, an incentive to dishonesty is built into transactions in which the realities of costs and consequences are so heavily disguised.

- *The capture of health services by producer interests and, within those interests, the domination of particular groups of providers.* Patients, in a public health service, are denied the strength which would be theirs within a more competitive market place. General practitioners are similarly disadvantaged in relation to hospital services, having to take what powerful providers will supply, rather than being able to influence that service by taking their custom elsewhere. Such a lack of responsiveness to consumers' preferences by monopoly public sector suppliers has been one of the major criticisms made against them by advocates of privatisation. In the health sector, the American academic, Enthoven (1985), who was to exercise a major influence over government thinking during the latter part of the 1980s, put it in this way: 'They are unresponsive to consumer preferences regarding times and places and modalities of treatment. They are guided much more by provider preferences and convenience than consumer preferences. They ration by queues. They lack accountability.'

- *The weak administration of health services, in which unproductive managers and administrators add to bureaucratic costs, without tackling the efficiency-distorting rewards of power and influence which accrued to status-hungry and authoritarian professionals in the medical setting.* Butcher (1995: 129) refers to health service managers in the NHS for more than thirty years after its foundation in 1948 as 'what Harrison (1988: 30) has described as "diplomats", concerned with minimising conflicts within the service and facilitating the work of the medical profession, rather than with attempting to bring about major change in the organisation and delivery of health care'. In the analysis of privatisers, 'diplomacy' and 'consensus' were weasel words, disguising weakness and inefficiency.

8.3 After 1979

The health service, in many ways, represented the greatest challenge for the free-marketeers who were progressively to dominate the Thatcher administrations of the 1980s. Here was an organisation which, in political terms, continued to command widespread affection and where the charge of 'privatisation' carried with it a real threat of political damage. For this reason, many commentators have portrayed the 1980s approach to health service reform as cautious, incremental and, until the very end of the decade, occupying a relatively peripheral part in government thinking. Pearson (1992: 215), for example, says 'the one "untouchable" which has thwarted the Thatcher government's mission to roll back the frontiers of the state has been the National Health Service'.

The argument of this chapter is somewhat different. It follows more closely the analysis suggested by the historian of the health service, Charles Webster (1998: 144) who suggests that for the ideologically committed members of the first Thatcher administration, 'the health service was regarded . . . as a prime test case for the assault on collectivism'. Despite a relatively innocuous 1979 Manifesto, the incoming Thatcher administration contained a collection of Ministers and policy advisers for whom reform of the health service was crucial. As he suggests (1998: 145),

> 'If the health service was not radically reformed, it would . . . block the crucial mission to roll back the state, reduce the scale of public expenditure, and expand the scope of the market economy . . . official advisers were eager to supply evidence concerning the offensiveness of Bevan's NHS to market and monetarist convictions. . . .
>
> 'The NHS was, therefore, a prime target for the ideologues of the right. . . . This radical agenda was by no means confined to an unrepresentative fringe . . . these objectives were characteristic of the aspirations of Mrs Thatcher's most trusted senior ministers and policy advisers.'

While the ideas which this group now pursued were already on the policy agenda before 1979, the spirit and scope with which such initiatives were now taken up was of a very different order from what had gone before. The areas to be considered here – managerialism, charging policies and private insurance – were explored and expanded against a continuous background of more radical reforming ideas proposed and promoted by Ministers and their policy advisers. Thus, for example, Maynard (1988: 47) suggests that, 'the report of the Central Policy Review Staff in September 1982 argued that one way by which the projected gap between government revenue and expenditure could be bridged was the denationalisation or "privatisation" of the National Health Service'. The efforts to push back the line of public provision, in the early 1980s, therefore took place on the back of a rapidly rising tide.

The account which follows begins with those elements which had already been apparent before 1979 but which, in the early 1980s, were transformed from marginal and tentative solutions – or those embarked upon as necessary evils – to essential and highly valued parts of a new strategy. It then goes on, in looking at the latter part of the decade, to consider those newer elements which emerged most strongly within health policy and which provided a distinctive character to the boundary shifts between private and public provision in this sector.

8.4 Developing old themes

Managerialism

Chapter 2 explored the general enthusiasm of the advocates of privatisation for private sector management techniques and approaches. In the health service, the 'consensus' management approach which had dominated its whole history was inevitably inimical to an administration whose leader was on record as dismissing the search for consensus within her own cabinet. In common with its approach in other policy areas, the government turned to a figure from outside the public sphere for advice. The resulting Griffiths Report of 1983 was sharply critical of consensus management, suggesting that, 'if Florence Nightingale were carrying her lamp through the corridors of the NHS today, she would almost certainly be searching for the people in charge'.

Griffiths recommended the appointment of general managers at the regional, district and unit levels within the health service. Butcher (1995: 131) describes the report, and the developments which followed it, as marking 'a radical change in the organisation and culture of health-care delivery'. The passive approach of public administration was to be replaced by the active and purposeful methods of the private sector. Within this new paradigm, power and influence swung sharply from medicine to management. Townsend *et al.* (1988: 25–6) identify two key shifts of principle which followed. Firstly, the new arrangements deposed the centrality of need in favour of efficiency. The internal workings of the health service – its use of resources, its management of personnel – were to be more important than the demands of 'the social context within which it is operating'. Secondly, the ethos of public administration, as well as its practice was diluted in the changes. Managerialism is not simply a set of techniques; it embodies, as Townsend *et al.* suggest, 'a set of beliefs about what was important and how things should be done'. And in the health service, the importance of public service and the primacy of the public good were on the wane. Webster (1998: 163–4) concludes that

> 'the profusion of management initiatives instituted during the first term of the Thatcher administration belies any claim that the government was diffident about confronting the existing culture of the NHS . . . Since the health service was not ripe for wholesale privat-isation, it seemed an ideal candidate for comprehensive application of the business methods associated with the New Public Management.'

Charging again

The founding principle of *free at the point of use* had been under pressure within the health service from the outset. From the early 1980s onwards, however, the substitution of private money for public through charging for services provided directly by the NHS, accelerated during this period. Prescription charges, which had been kept at 20p an item during the 1970s, were raised to £1 per item in December 1980. Within ten years, the cost of a prescription in real terms had risen by some 500 per cent. The practical effect of these changes, according to Powell (1996: 36), was that 'many people now find it cheaper to buy their prescriptions over the counter. In other words, a process of re-commodification appears to be occurring.'

New charges for ophthalmic and dental services were announced in 1987, followed, two years later, by the abolition, other than for exempted groups, of free dental checks and free eye tests. At the same time, the age limit for free dental treatment was reduced from 21 to 16. Webster (1998: 158) estimates that 'as a consequence of restriction . . . there was an immediate reduction by two-thirds in the number of sight tests, and a fall of more than half in spectacles supplied under the NHS'. By 1996 the *Health Service Journal* reported that more than a million NHS patients had been deregistered by dentists since 1992. Further changes introduced by the government then required patients to attend for a dental check-up every fifteen months or face automatic removal from the dental register. This change led to 4.1 million people being removed from NHS dentistry lists during 1996 (*The Independent* 15 August 1997). By the end of that year, only 52 per cent of the population were registered with the NHS dentistry service. Levenson's (1992: 28) prediction that 'NHS dentistry is on its way to becoming an endangered species' had proved to be correct. As he suggested, for the general population, it now appeared 'to be more in the realm of the market than part of the NHS'.

In addition to the more headline-grabbing methods of generating additional funding from private sources a series of other measures, instituted during the 1980s, were designed to increase the flow of revenue to the health service from individuals rather than the Exchequer. Butler (1993: 56) summarises the approach to charging in this way:

> 'The promise was held out of a future replete with commercial potential: among the things that might be considered suitable for sale were clinical services, expertise, amenity beds, laboratory services, catering services, advertising space, car parking slots and conference facilities . . . Shopping arcades could be built in unfilled corridors and health clubs opened in unused basements. Mail order services were created to sell everything from bandages to stretchers, and fees were charged for measuring the bodies of those who died in hospital.'

The practical effect of such initiatives was considerable. The 1980 Health Services Act allowed health authorities to organise appeals and to use Exchequer funds for this purpose. Hundreds of appeals followed and funds available to health authorities from charitable-giving increased from £57 million in 1985/86 to £220 million in 1990/91 (Ruane 1997: 55). Investment of income on a short-term basis between payment for and delivery of services, raised £70m in 1993/94.

The extension of charges in the post-1979 period continued to have the greatest impact upon those who were neither exempt from them, nor sufficiently well-off to be able to pay without difficulty. Birch (1986), for example, shows that the increase in prescription charges led to a fall in take-up rates for those in the non-exempt group. Nor were cost-savings automatically generated by the new techniques. Goldsmith (1997: 17), writing as the Vice Chairman of the Conservative Medical Society – a specialist policy adviser to successive Secretaries of State for Health and intimately involved in the development of the 1990 NHS reforms – concluded that the introduction of dental and eye charges 'have actually been damaging both to the government's reputation and probably to the patients' health. In particular this is true of the abolition of free eye-tests . . . Recent research has shown that rates of untreated glaucoma may actually have risen because of the disincentive to preventative eye care caused by the charges.'

Even in its own terms, then, transferring costs from the collective to the individual may not have lived up to the claims made by privatisation enthusiasts. In health care, the avoidance of costs at one level may simply lead to the postponement of costs at a higher personal and financial level, rather than their elimination. The claim that private responsibility would drive out public inefficiency is not borne out, even where costs are most directly reallocated between the one and the other.

Private health care

Advocates of choice and diversity in health care had long pointed to the absence of a level playing field, as they regarded it, between the monolithic NHS and the far smaller private health care market. It was a natural approach, for a government dedicated to the advantage of private provision, to set about encouraging the growth of private health insurance. Here was a sector which would provide choice between public and private and, by operating in a competitive environment, would deliver the benefits of consumer sovereignty and price restraint. As a result, as Butcher (1995: 113) summarises: 'The private health care sector underwent tremendous changes in the 1980s: the percentage of the UK population covered by private health insurance more than trebled between 1979 and 1989. There was also a rapid growth of private hospitals, the private sector's share of hospital-based health care in the UK doubling between 1984 and 1990' (Baggott 1994: 153, 156).

Free marketeers often suggest that government intervention should be limited to clearing the ring, removing their own interference and allowing the forces of enterprise a free rein. In the health case, however, as Mohan (1986: 41) points out, the rise of the private sector has at least as much to do with the highly visible hand of the government as with the hidden hand of the market. The growth in private medicine has been directly encouraged, for example, by planning decisions, changes in consultants' contracts and tax on medical insurance premiums. Just as in the case of private rented housing, tax concessions to providers, as well as consumers of private health care, were influential in creating the market. According to Pearson (1992: 222),

'Other measures promoting small business during Thatcher's first term encouraged the growth of the private sector. The Business Start-up Scheme and Business Expansion Scheme, introduced in the 1981 budget, offered tax concessions against expenses incurred in creating or expanding small business. Consultants used these provisions to set up their own private hospitals.'

As a result, by the time of the fiftieth anniversary of the NHS, Webster (1998: 154–6) suggests that 'consortiums of private providers and NHS consultants acting in their private capacity were colonising many services which had hitherto been entirely the province of the NHS'. Figures provided by Pearson (1992: 222) translate this effort into beds and expenditure. In his estimation, 'between 1979 and 1985, the number of beds in private hospitals in the UK increased by 54 per cent to 10,155. Private spending on health care increased by 456 per cent between 1978 and 1988, compared with an increase of 195 per cent in NHS expenditure.'

This substantial change was not brought about solely by the preference for an insurance-based approach to paying for health care. Ruane (1997: 57) points to a series of other ways in which, over this period, the interface between private and public sectors in health care was made more permeable, to the advantage of the private sector. Changes in the 1988 Health and Medicines Act resulted in an increase in pay-bed income for trusts from £32.2 million in 1991/92 to £115 million in 1993/94. Ruane concludes that the NHS increased its shared of the private acute market to 16 per cent over the same period while noting that 'the other side of the coin concerns the extent of health-care for NHS patients provided by the private sector. Health authorities have been able since 1981 to place contracts with commercial hospitals . . . Parliamentary figures suggest that NHS spending on private care rose by almost 170 per cent between 1991/2 and 1994/5 to £850 million'.

As in the case of managerialism and charging policies, the encouragement of private health provision embodies a series of ethical as well as practical consequences. Powell (1996: 37), for example, concludes that the claim to *comprehensiveness* made by the NHS was 'undermined in the 1980s as many people took the exit option from the NHS and went private, joining the queue where rationing is by money rather than by need'.

Allsop (1997: 12) draws out the consequences of private insurance-based health care for the principle of equity in health care. Her summary succinctly draws together a series of key arguments and is worth quoting in full:

'Compared to collective ownership, in a market system of health care, private capital inevitably seeks profit. Private suppliers are likely to avoid high cost, specialist care where there is low demand but where there is a high research and development cost. Neither can the private sector be expected to be committed to ensuring national coverage or equity in access and outcome. On the demand side, user charges deter people seeking medical attention, even if there is a clinical need. Private insurance, in the economist's term, "skims cream". It selects the best risks – that is, the healthiest – and often limits cover to exclude high cost care. Under such a system inequities in the distribution of health care and the differences in health care outcomes would be likely to increase. Moreover, market forces tend to operate to fulfil short-term individual wants rather than long-term investment in the collective interest.'

As earlier chapters have suggested, the case for privatisation in social policy areas rests upon a variety of claims, not all of which might be fulfilled in any particular instance. If private health provision fails a test of equity, it might, nonetheless, provide substantial benefits in relation to economy or efficiency. Yet, it seems clear that the absence of any direct connection between money paid and service delivered provides as great a difficulty – as viewed by privatisers – in the case of private insurance as the public health service. As Maynard (1988: 52) suggests, 'the patient, whether public or private, is provided with care at zero price and has little incentive to minimise costs because, after all, the third party (NHS or BUPA) pays!' Indeed, far from cost-minimisation, the charges made by private health companies rose faster than the retail price index during the 1980s, moving ahead at an average of between 6 and 12 per cent each year above inflation.

Without equity or efficiency, the benefits of choice and consumer preference remain the strongest claim to be made for private health care. Yet, even here, by the mid-1990s, concern about the operation of the private health care market had led to an inquiry by the Office of Fair Trading. Far from confirming the claims made by the advocates of free-markets, the ensuing report (OFT 1996) showed that: 'The combination of medical matters and insurance makes these products doubly difficult to understand and almost impossible to compare.' The market, far from promoting choice and diversity, had produced circumstances in which it was 'difficult for even the well educated to make good judgements'. As Ranade (1997: 84) points out, such circumstances fail to provide any 'true test of the New Right model of suppliers reacting directly to consumer preferences in the market-place'.

This chapter has been concerned, to this point, with the development of ways of redressing the public–private boundary in health care which, essentially, picked up and gave substantial new impetus to ideas which had been present, in one form or another, throughout the history of the health service. It now moves on to consider three more radical departures which were far more the creatures and creations of their own time: contacting out of services, the redefinition of medical and social care and the creation of an internal market within the health service.

8.5 Creating new approaches

Contracting out

Of the three areas to be considered in this section, contracting out is most firmly based upon the central principle of privatisation, that the primary responsibility of public organisations lies in ensuring the availability rather than the direct provision of services. Many of the services provided directly by the NHS, it was argued, could be provided by the private sector, providing the advantages of efficiency, innovation and customer-sensitivity. The in-coming government of 1979 faced a situation in which only some 2 per cent of the spending on support services was made in the private sector. In 1983 a DHSS circular aimed to alter this situation. It instructed health authorities to put the three hospital ancillary services of cleaning, laundry and catering (the so-called 'hotel services') out to competitive tender. From 1987 onwards the process spread steadily, beginning with other non-clinical services (such as portering, transport and computing), but, as Butler (1993) makes clear, thereafter

'it quickly spread to quasi-clinical services (such as sterile supplies) and then to clinical services (such as pathology). By the end of 1990, a directory of business opportunities in the NHS was reportedly in circulation, detailing commercial possibilities in such areas as pathology, blood transfusion services, information technology, property development and retailing.'

Despite these considerable efforts, the practical impact of competitive tendering and contracting out within the health service was less dramatic than such a list might suggest. Butcher (1995: 112), for example, concludes that 'CCT has had only limited success in transferring these services to the private sector, as the majority of contracts have been won by in-house tenders. Thus, by the end of 1991, only 14 per cent of contracts in the three ancillary services had been awarded to private companies.' Yet, the price of winning contacts in-house was often high. Competing on cost depended upon driving down both wages and staff numbers. In the process, quality of service – which private sector involvement was meant to enhance – suffered. In the argument presented in this book, therefore, the costs savings which privatisation brought, were achieved by cost-creation elsewhere. The savings in the public sphere were the product of the private consequences left in the lives of some of the poorest paid workers in the public service and in the taxpayer's bill for the unemployment which followed.

Social care and medical care

If contracting out of ancillary services represents a significant shift in health service operations, the second area to be considered in this section carried some of the same techniques and arguments far further. Chapter 7 dealt in more detail with the impact upon social services departments of the redefinition of 'medical' and 'social' care. Here that process can be viewed as part of the general effort to 'contract out' those elements of activity which might be removed from the account of one organisation and placed in that of another. For the most part, but by no means exclusively, the impact of this change is felt among older people whose conditions are chronic and unlikely to respond to treatment.

As Chapters 5 and 7 have demonstrated, the social security changes of the 1980s produced an explosion in the private residential care sector for older people. If the availability of such help provided the 'pull', then the 'push' came from managers of hospitals, freeing up their own budgets by transferring long-stay patients to the DSS-funded private care sector. Thus, as Ranade (1997: 206) suggests, 'even before the NHS and Community Care Act 1990 health authorities had started to define the long-stay care of elderly people as "not part of our core business"'. The 1990 Act provided new impetus to policies already well developed within the health sphere.

The impact of these changes, however, was felt well beyond those conditions which appeared unamenable to treatment and outside the narrowly curative remit which market players wished to create for themselves. Ruane (1997: 58) identifies a series of other settings in which NHS treatment might be denied:

> 'Older people face refusal of access to Accident and Emergency Units as well as discharge to nursing homes in the event of terminal illness on the basis that they have no clinical reason to occupy a hospital bed. This erosion of access to free health-care applies not only to long-term and chronic conditions, but increasingly to complex and acute conditions.'

The redefinition of what counts as available health care is fundamental to the privatisation project on a number of counts. At the cost level, it substitutes free medical care by means-tested social care, a shift which, for the group most affected, has been described by Powell (1996: 38) as 'essentially moving the goalposts after the taxpaying horse has been put out to pasture'. Of course, costs themselves do not disappear; they fall either to other budgets – such as social security or social services – or upon the savings and other resources of individuals themselves. In this shift, not only are direct costs transferred from public to private but the responsibility for care in later life is similarly altered. The state no longer accepts the obligations which it had previously undertaken for the welfare of some of its most vulnerable citizens, leaving that burden to be met, as best it might, in the lives of those most directly affected.

Competition, the internal market and 'Working for Patients'

In January 1988, Mrs Thatcher appeared on television and, to the surprise of commentators and her own supporters – including those in the Cabinet (Maynard 1995) – announced a hitherto untrailed review. According to Butler (1993: 60–1), 'the review . . . took exactly a year to complete, was conducted in private by a small group of cabinet ministers, chaired by Mrs Thatcher herself. . . . By the summer of 1988 . . . attention began to deflect away from the volume and sources of money going into the NHS towards the ways in which it is used.' The 'internal market', as it came to be known, was to be the device through which that radical reframing of the use of resources was be achieved. The text of the White Paper, *Working for Patients*, which followed described this as 'a funding system in which successful hospitals can flourish . . . will encourage greater competition. All this in turn will ensure a better deal for the public, improving the choice and quality of services offered and the efficiency with which these services are delivered' (DoH 1989: 22).

While the White Paper usefully emphasised the objectives of the internal market – increased efficiency, enhanced consumer choice and improved quality of service – it completely ignored, as Hunter (1997: 48) points out, 'the source of the problem – alleged underfunding'. Drawing clearly on the advice of Allain Enthoven, who proposed an internal market within the NHS in which providers of services would compete with each other for funds, the 1990 National

Health Service and Community Care Act instituted a separation between the responsibility for the purchase of services (demand) from their delivery (supply). On the demand side, individual patients were not to be provided directly with purchasing rights. Rather, three different categories of budget-holder were to act as agents, purchasing services on their behalf. They were to be the main purchasing authority – the District Health Authority – the budget-holding general practitioner, and the private sector, primarily through insurers. On the supply side, services would be provided by those hospitals which remained under the direct management of health authorities, or by self-governing NHS trusts which had opted out of health authority control, supplemented by private and voluntary providers. In this explicit preference for market over planning, the White Paper appeared to the considerable majority of those associated with the health service as, in the words of Butler (1993: 56), to 'finally mark the break with the service structures erected by Bevan and Beveridge'.

It cannot be part of this chapter's purpose to provide a detailed account of the introduction and development of the internal market in the health service and a number of excellent accounts of these changes already exist (e.g. Allsop 1995; Ranade 1997). However, briefly, the provider role within the new system developed more rapidly than originally anticipated. The first wave of 57 independent trusts came into being on the first day of the new arrangements, in April 1991, accounting for 13.5 per cent of NHS revenue expenditure. As Smee (1995: 181) records, by the time the fourth wave became operational in April 1994, this had increased to 95 per cent.

The purchasing side, by contrast, developed more slowly. In the first instance, faced again with an imminent general election, the government insisted that a 'steady state' be maintained in which the major purchasers, the District Health Authorities, were instructed to maintain a flow of funds to providers on the basis of historical patterns of service delivery. At the micro-purchasing level, however, change was more rapid. Substantial financial inducements for participation, together with a sequential lowering of the number of patients needed by a practice in order to qualify, led to an increase in the number of GP fundholders to a point where, according to a 1996 Audit Commission Report, half the population were now covered in this way (Audit Commission 1996). Here, individual doctors were both purchasers of services from hospital suppliers and themselves encouraged to develop a more competitive market as suppliers of primary health care. As Ranade (1997: 72) explains, the remuneration system for GPs was used to encourage this way of working, 'by increasing the proportion of the GP's income derived from capitation fees from the average of 45 per cent to 60 per cent, GPs were encouraged to "compete" for more patients by offering higher standards of care'.

With the Conservative victory of 1992, the thrust towards marketisation gathered pace. Butler (1993: 68) suggests that 'managers who succeeded in retaining their jobs in the tense political climate enjoyed a field-day of unprecedented freedom to review their alliances, extend their fiefdoms and generally rewrite the rules of the game to their own advantage'.

The period of the Major administration concentrated upon consolidating the reforms of *Working for Patients* and carrying the market processes further. The most significant new feature was provided by the Private Finance Initiative in which NHS facilities were developed by private capital in conjunction with an NHS partner *[document 6]*. At the end of the process the physical products were owned by the contractor and leased back to the health service. Direct provision of services, other than those covered by a contracting definition of 'clinical', could also be provided by the same private contractor. The development of the PFI was slower and more cumbersome than its privatisation supporters had suggested. There were 57 such projects in different stages of operation by August 1996, at a value of some £500 million. By the time of the 1997 General Election a number of themes had emerged.

Firstly, at primary care level, the increasing number of fundholding practitioners produced persistent criticisms that a 'two-tier' system had been created, in which fundholders were able to purchase a better level of care for their patients, potentially at the expense of those in greater clinical need. The mechanism which produced this critique was simple. Any additional fundholding budget meant a corresponding reduction in the budget of the District Health Authority from which emergency services for all, and other services for non-fundholders had to be provided. According to Webster (1998: 200), the result risked the production of 'a residual service for the poorer sections of the community'.

Secondly, the practical business of competition appeared to be at risk of providing a series of disbenefits. The organisation of the annual contracting round proved both time-consuming and one in which rewards were incommensurate with the costs – financial and human – which the process entailed. 'Success' in one area, moreover, could lead to perverse consequences in others with, for example, faster hospital discharges producing extra burdens for GPs having to deal with 'more patients discharged from hospital "quicker and sicker"' Ranade (1997: 210).

Thirdly, the whole concept of 'competition' proved to be more elusive in practice than in the model from which it was derived. North (1998: 7), in one of the early detailed investigations of the new health market in action, notes that 'advice from the Department of Health was unequivocal in its attempts to forestall price cartels and other forms of provider collusion . . . the regulatory effort invested in maintaining a degree of contestability in local markets is testimony to its considered importance'. In the study, which investigated the purchasing strategies of one DHA in its relationship with an acute and community-based trust, the power in the new market arrangements was assumed to lie with the purchaser. The income of hospital and community trusts now depended upon contracts won from GP fundholders and health authorities, and failure to obtain such contracts would lead to market failure. In practice, however, the purchasing health authority failed to make the progress which such a powerful starting point might have suggested. The authority began with what North (1998: 12–13) describes as a 'misplaced confidence in the threat of a contestable market' and proceeded to attempt to engender a competitive milieu by treating all potential providers on a strictly equal basis, as required by free market tenets. The result was a rupturing of relationships with local providers, and what North calls 'a mirage of competition' which did not, in fact, attract any alternative providers. The upshot was a failure to implement the strategy which the purchaser had carefully drawn up and embarked upon. North's conclusion (1998: 13) is telling. He identifies the over-confidence of the purchaser in its market power, at the expense of an appreciation of the importance of reciprocity, trust and co-operation, even in commercial markets. 'Paradoxically,' he concludes 'it was the very artificiality of the local market in health care and the need to maintain the impression of competitiveness in purchaser–provider relationships which proved so disruptive.' Hunter (1997: 51) draws the more general conclusion that:

> 'The marketisation of health care has eroded "high-trust" relationships. Trust implies mutual understanding and respect. Whatever its short-comings, the pre-1984 NHS was based on "high-trust" relationships in which the parties involved observed mutual obligations which were not precisely defined. The post-1984 and 1991 changes introduced relationships which imply low trust: everything must be defined, documented, formalised and transformed into a quasi-contractual relationship.'

The 'new economic sociology' (Grantovetter and Swedberg 1992) has drawn out the economic implications of the tensions between the competitive conditions of pure markets and the trust relationships of social welfare contracts. While trust is the product of social relationships, it has important economic consequences in contributing to decision making. Mannion and Smith (1998: 130) put it in this way: 'Trust within this context serves as a lubricant of economic exchanges by reducing the transaction costs associated with regulating the quasi-market. It operates as an intangible capital asset which economises on the costs of bargaining, monitoring, insurance and dispute settlement.'

Even before the Conservative period in office ended in May 1997, Webster (1998) concludes that the early phases of the internal market were tending away from the contracting culture in at least two important ways. Firstly, the Humpty Dumpty plethora of small and competing units, into which the advocates of privatisation had carefully broken up the monolithic structures which so offended them within the NHS, were soon busily trying to put themselves back together again. As Ranade (1997: 96) suggests, these tendencies were part of a wider pattern of commercial life: 'Although the introduction of the quasi-market was intended to replace planning (certainty) by market forces (uncertainty), uncertainty was the one characteristic of markets which they themselves try to overcome by the creation of cartels or monopolies.' Thus, the fierce competitors of the market imagination were turning tame. Mutual dependence and the operational efficiency of trust-based practice was leading, as Webster (1998: 200) put it, to 'a revival of a consensual approach to decision-making at the heart of health-service resource management'.

8.6 Assessing the reforms

The various reforms reviewed in this chapter have the cumulative effect of transforming what Ranade describes as the 'creeping privatisation' of the 1980s into a policy which, in practice, had captured much of the high ground and which, in Webster's (1998: 141) words, 'amounted to a continuous revolution, which brought about a profound transformation in the culture of the NHS'. It is against this background that an assessment of the claims made for the reforms must be made. One of the enduring themes of privatisation advocates suggests that a shift in this direction would produce gains in efficiency, economy, choice, accountability and responsiveness, while maintaining the principle of equity [document 5]. Some verdicts upon these claims have already been suggested at earlier points in this chapter. Some brief assessment in relation to each one now follows.

Efficiency

Attacks on inefficiency in health service administration are commonplace in the discourses of political parties, and had found a prominent place in the Conservative Manifesto of 1979. Yet, costs within the public health service have always been far lower than those that can be achieved within alternative insurance-based or purely private provision. Maynard (1995: 80) puts it in this way: 'The NHS has been cheap to administer – less than 5 per cent of total costs were spent on NHS management in the NHS in the 1980s, compared to in excess of 15 per cent in the USA and in the UK private sector.'

The internal market reforms, in particular, soon imported private sector practices into the public sphere, even though, as Morgan (1995: 2) suggests, the strong presumption that private sector management practices were superior to those of the public sector was 'seldom challenged or subjected to critical testing'. While beds were closed and staff levels fell, the number of administrators and clerical officers in the NHS rose by 18 per cent between 1981 and 1991 and by a further 10 per cent thereafter. The growth in senior managers, as demanded by the new managerialist culture, was even more spectacular. Webster (1998: 203) reports that in England just under 1,000 individuals were classed as general or senior managers in 1986, rising to 16,000 in 1991 and 26,000 in 1995. Nor were all these posts applied at a cerebrally cutting edge. As Ham (1994: 296) suggests: 'Management in the NHS has come to resemble a paper chase as NHS trusts seek to secure their income by negotiating with different purchasers and as all players in the market invest in information systems to monitor contract compliance.' Maynard (1995: 71) puts the costs, in the first few years of the reforms, at an additional £1,000 million spent on information technology and increased managerial requirements, concluding that 'the cost-effectiveness of this expenditure is as unknown as the opportunity cost (in terms of patient care) is obvious'.

By 1997, the inefficiency and bureaucracy of the new style health service had come to play as prominent a part in the New Labour Manifesto as it had ever filled in the same document produced by the Conservatives almost twenty years before.

Economy

Nor do the cost arguments stand up to close scrutiny. As Maynard (1995: 71) suggests:

'The fragmentation of all health-care systems creates incentives for cash-limited decision-makers to shift patients and hence costs from their budgets to those of other component parts of the health-care system. Thus in the NHS a manager with a cash-limited hospital system may shift drug costs on to the primary-care system. With the hospital buying in bulk and using cheap generic drugs and the primary-care GP prescribing expensive brand-named drugs, this behaviour may increase the NHS drugs bill with no significant benefits in patient outcome.'

Choice

The emphasis which supporters of privatisation in social welfare services place upon the question of choice emerges, on closer inspection, to be both contra-dictory and internally inconsistent. Indeed, as Maynard (1988: 51) puts it, 'the market for health care is inherently uncertain. The patient–consumer does not know when he will be ill and when illness strikes he will be uncertain as to diagnosis and treatment.' Indeed, he goes on to suggest that: 'The nature of the health care market, especially the uncertainty inherent in diagnosis and treat-ment, is such that competition may lead to harm to individuals in society.'

Against this uncertain background, many of the market claims lack sustain-ability because these are not proper markets: purchasers lack proper informa-tion; individuals do not have power of purchase, having that exercised for them through surrogates – a situation which Webster (1998: 202) describes as 'not so much a matter of the patient dictating where the money went, but the patient following whatever channel the professionals dictated'. As noted in the example provided by North (1998) above, moreover, local hospitals are often monopoly providers and make real competition impossible. The argument of market sup-porters has to rely upon the weaker ground of 'contestability', i.e. that there could be competition, potentially, and that this would influence the behaviour of local monopolists. Yet, as already demonstrated, contestability in practice has turned out to be a misleading guide to action, sowing dissension and distrust among real providers in order to play them off against potential suppliers who were never likely to materialise.

Accountability

For free marketeers, accountability exists in the relationship between suppliers and customers, with individuals exercising their influence as consumers rather than as citizens. Yet, in practice, such users have little direct power within the health service. At a managerial level, those acting on their behalf are often not engaged on a day-by-day basis with the delivery of services. As Roberts *et al.*

(1998: 284) conclude, 'this distancing of contractors from the users of services is a problem common to many quasi-markets'. Wall (1996: 76) has investigated the operation of accountability within the health service internal market. He found that 'the reluctance of the large majority of health authorities and trusts to hold their meetings in public, [is] one of the simpler tests for accountability'. In the new competitive conditions, claims to commercial confidentiality were advanced to exclude the public from an ever-widening circle of subjects. At an individual level, also, Wall (1996: 82) suggests that the very processes of the internal market contribute not to enhanced accountability or transparency, as the supporters of privatisation claim, but lead to buckpassing and confusion in which the division between purchaser and provider allows individuals and organisations to escape the responsibility for their own actions, always providing someone else to blame when things go wrong. 'In such a system', he concludes, 'accountability will never fully operate.'

Equity

Finally, to turn to the question of equity – the claim which, as this book has consistently demonstrated, causes the greatest of difficulties for the advocates of privatisation. This is especially acute in the case of health where, as Robinson (1988) suggests, considerable importance has traditionally been attached to equity outcomes. Broadly following his analysis, three sets of arguments suggest that, in a market, the distribution of services is likely to be more unequal than in the system it had replaced.

Firstly, in any market, income and the ability to pay will become the major determinant of access to goods and services. Purchase of services is related to income; supply of services is shaped by the need to extract an income. This chapter has traced a series of ways in which costs previously met within the health service have been transferred to the individual. Ability to pay, rather than need, inevitably becomes the major factor which determines outcomes in this situation.

Secondly, organisations which have to maximise income or cut-back on costs are always likely to take into their calculations the income-generating potential of particular treatments of groups of patients on the one hand, and the resource demands of other groups and treatments on the other. Whitehead (1994), for example, has argued that 'providers have an inbuilt incentive to concentrate on serving more prosperous and healthy populations at the expense of those patients with chronic conditions, who are more expensive to treat'. This chapter has already added to the cumulative evidence that, in any market, the creation of winners meets its inevitable counterpart in the creation of losers. The 1997/98 Report of the Health Service Ombudsman (Health Service Commissioner 1998: 10–11) highlighted concern at the actions of family doctors striking patients off their lists without explanation or 'common courtesy'. The Report concluded that 'some GPs too readily regard the fact that a complaint has been made as sufficient evidence that the doctor–patient relationship has broken down'. Patients, for their part, were likely to be 'inhibited by fear' from making a complaint, if removal from their GP's list were to be the consequence. In the argument of this book, the increasing difficulties identified in the report are an inevitable, rather than unintended, consequence of marketisation.

Thirdly, and more specifically, the GP fundholder initiative has been criticised for the greater inequity that has resulted. The discussion returns us to one of the core claims of privatisation enthusiasts with which this chapter began – that is, the claim that socialised medicine represented an unacceptable diminution in the freedom of the individual which markets would put right. The freedom of GP fundholders to obtain a better deal for their patients, however, has been achieved at the expense of non-fundholder patients. According to Ahmed (1996: 88):

'The reforms have posed a challenge to equity in that GPFHs patients in many parts of the country have been able to secure quicker access to hospitals than other patients. Given the concentration of GPFHs in more affluent parts of the country, this has served to accentuate Tudor-Hart's law of inverse care which states that access to good medical care is most available where it is least needed.'

8.7 Summary

The level of political support for the National Health Service provided a level of challenge to the privatising enterprise which was unrivalled in other social welfare services. As such, it has led some commentators to suggest that neo-liberal prescriptions were applied only tentatively in this area, and with only superficial results. The argument of this chapter has been different. Caution in political presentation did not prevent successive attempts to alter the balance between private and public responsibilities in relation to health at an individual and structural level. By the end of the period of Conservative administration in 1997, the National Health Service was dominated by features of a market system to an extent which would have been quite unthinkable in 1979. The benefits which such alterations were intended to deliver, however, had risen considerably less conspicuously than the tide of enthusiasm upon which they had been introduced.

The last word, in assessing the reforms of the 1980s and 1990s, may be left to Webster (1998: 204) who concludes thus:

'The internal-market reforms compare unfavourably with the discredited "command economy" structure introduced in 1948, for which considerably bolder claims could be made about the advances in output, performance, consumer satisfaction, and morale of health-service personnel.'

PART THREE

Chapter 9

HOUSING, SOCIAL SECURITY AND EDUCATION AFTER 1997

The first Labour government for nearly 20 years was elected on 1 May 1997. This chapter, and the one which follows, provides an account of the actions of that government in key social policy areas, investigating once again the ways in which such policies address the fundamental boundary between public and private responsibility.

The current chapter concentrates upon the areas of housing, social security and education. Chapter 10 will deal with social services and health policies and attempt some general overview of patterns which emerge across the social policy agenda.

9.1 Housing

As Chapter 4 suggested, the legacy of Conservative government in housing was profound, to the extent that some commentators (see, for example, Glennerster and Hills 1998) suggested that it had ceased to be an area of policy development in its own right. It had become instead an adjunct to other disciplines and administrative responsibilities, driven along by decisions made in the fields of social security and urban regeneration. Early in the new administration, Ministers moved to suggest that housing would occupy a very different place in political priorities. The new Housing Minister, Hilary Armstrong, told the Annual Conference of the Chartered Institute of Housing on 27 June 1997 that 'housing is at the very heart of society' and would occupy a 'key role' in the government's social policy agenda (DETR 1997a). The Deputy Prime Minister, John Prescott, similarly emphasised the core contribution which local authority services, through housing and education, would make to the achievement of social justice (DETR 1997b).

Within six months of taking office, the basic approach of the new administration to housing matters was set out by the Minister responsible, Hilary Armstrong, in an address to the annual Conference of the National Housing Federations. 'I am not interested', said the Minister, 'in housing ideologies; I am interested in what works' (DETR 1997c). She was, she told delegates, 'open-minded' about solutions, which needed to include a 'healthy private sector' as well as local authority and social housing. Agnosticism about ideology is a theme which was to be repeated in other social policy areas after May 1997. Doing 'what works' included both a new belief in the power of the state to effect change in people's lives and in the contribution of the market. This contribution formed the centre-piece of the Minister's speech to the Chartered Institute of Housing (DETR 1998a), 12 months into the new government, when she set out to define the administration's approach to the scope and nature of government intervention in the housing field. Of the housing market, she declared that:

> 'Our overriding aim is to make the housing market work for all the people. If the housing market worked perfectly there would be no need or rationale for government interven-tion, but the free market cannot accommodate the needs and aspirations of all. Govern-ment must intervene, but that intervention must be limited and strategic.'

In comparison with the free marketeers of the previous decade, this state-ment clearly draws a new set of policy imperatives. Markets were important, but characterised by significant limitations, particularly in relation to equity. Public intervention in market processes was therefore justifiable when outcomes required modification. The market remained the essential mechanism by which the demand and supply of housing was to be reconciled, but a market shaped by government intervention, 'to make the market work for all the people, pro-tect the vulnerable and reduce the scope for exploitation'.

The brief account which now follows considers the practical application of this new approach to a series of housing policy areas. Following the pattern adopted in the concluding section of Chapter 4, these are grouped around the impact produced by policies upon those who buy their own homes, those in the rented sector and those without a home at all. A final section will deal briefly with the effect on housing of the Comprehensive Spending Review.

People who buy their own homes

One of the earliest concessions made by Labour in opposition to the privatisa-tion agenda had come with its conversion to the policy of selling council houses. By May 1997, the high-water mark of that policy was well past, but continued to enjoy the support of the new administration. In line with its tendency to intervene in order to level the market playing field, however, the government also announced, in July 1998, its intention to consult on 'changing discounts to purchasers under the Right to Buy scheme, to ensure the scheme gives the taxpayer better value for money' (DETR 1998b).

More generally, the state of crisis which had characterised the owner-occupied housing market during the early 1990s was at an end by May 1997. The number of house repossessions was in decline during the middle years of the decade but began to rise again in 1998. Home repossessions increased in the first six months of 1998 by 10 per cent over the previous six months, with 600 people a week losing their homes. The Lord Chancellor's department figures showed repossession actions up 19 per cent on the same time in 1997 (*The Guardian* 30.7.98 and 19.10.98). In this field, however, the new government looked to the same set of solutions as its predecessors. In opposition, Labour had published plans to combine fixed-term private mortgage insurance with state cover for those out of work for over a year (*The Times* 17.9.96). In office, the first budget of the new government lowered MIRAS from 15 to 10 per cent and proved unreceptive to proposals to develop a social security benefit for low-income households purchasing their own homes by mortgage. Instead, and despite evidence of the unsatisfactory outcomes – see Chapter 4 – the government preferred to rely upon market solutions, looking to lenders and insurers to provide better protection (*The Times* 9.9.97).

Those who remain in the rented sector

In relation to demand for rented housing, the incoming administration took early steps to reverse the previous government's intentions to cut housing benefit by extending the 'single room rent' rule to people aged 25–59. It was, suggested Deakin and Parry (1998: 43), 'the one major reversal' in the so-called 'Lilley overhang' of policies inherited from the previous administration. The limit remained in place for those aged below 25, despite evidence that landlords were refusing to rent to young people because of benefit cuts (Shelter 1998). The money which would have been saved through an extension of the single room rent rule was recovered, instead, by an increase in the rate of non-dependent deduction from housing benefit and reducing the time limit during which claims for the benefit could be backdated from three months to one month.

In relation to supply, Labour inherited the promotion of private renting which had been a traditional aim of Conservative administrations. During the 1980s and 1990s this had been underpinned by reductions in protection offered to tenants and, latterly, by direct financial incentives through the tax concessions in Housing Investment Trusts. Labour's Housing Minister, Hilary Armstrong, soon made it clear to the sector that these advantages would go unchanged. She told the Association of Residential Letting Agents (DETR 1997d) that the Government had absolutely 'no plans to change the established framework of assured and assured-shorthold tenancies. We will maintain our support for the concept of Housing Investment Trusts. We welcome initiatives to encourage and support the growth of responsible letting.'

It was the supply side of public housing, however, which had been the most strongly trailed element in Labour's policy during the run-up to the 1997 General Election. Indeed, the release of capital receipts built up by local authorities through the sale of council houses was one of the few direct commitments to additional public spending with which the Party entered the election period. The task faced was a formidable one. The National Housing Forum (1997) published a report early in 1997 which suggested that 1.65 million homes in England and Wales were unfit for human habitation, and a further 95,000 in Scotland were 'below the tolerable standard'. The final Conservative budget, meanwhile, had cut local authority funds for housing improvement by £200 million. A start on the implementation of Labour's policy began in its first

Budget which took place within weeks of assuming office. Specific proposals for a Capital Receipts Initiative were announced on 19 June 1997, emphasising the priority of targeting additional resources on housing and housing-related regeneration schemes and making proposals for distributing resources between local authorities. The first budget of the new administration announced the release of £200 million in 1997/98, followed by a further £700 million in 1998/99 (DETR 1997e).

At the same time, the Government moved to address the additional revenue costs through interest charges, or reduced interest on the investment of receipts, created by increased capital investment. Extra support was provided to local authorities investing in council housing under the Capital Receipts Initiative, in a further example of the new administration's positive belief in the benefits of directed public expenditure. In contradistinction to the policies of the previous government, the same revenue settlement also limited rent increases in the public housing sector to an average of 97p a week, and was accompanied by a ministerial exhortation to councils to 'keep rent increases down' (DETR 1997f).

The second strand in the new administration's approach to the public rented sector showed far greater affiliation with the policies of its predecessor. By the time Labour took up office there were more than 2,200 Registered Social Landlords, as housing associations were now known, owning some 856,000 homes and providing 70,000 hostel places. To a significant extent, as Chapter 4 demonstrated, the growth in the sector had been the result of large-scale voluntary transfer of council housing stock. From the local authority perspective this had been driven by the resulting capital receipts and, from central government by the level of private finance which it now required in social landlord schemes. Under Labour, these initiatives were enthusiastically continued and developed. By February 1998, for example, 63 local authorities had transferred their stock to housing associations, involving 252,000 dwellings, £2.5 billion in capital receipts and over £4 billion in private finance (DETR 1998c). Five of these transactions, involving 18,000 dwellings valued at over £160 million, took place during the first year of Labour Government. In March 1998 the Department announced a possible further 28 transfers which, the Minister said, 'reflects the Government's commitment to a continuing programme of transfers as a means of generating private finance' (DETR 1998d).

Sixteen of the 28 potential transfers were to be brought about with assistance from the Estates Renewal Challenge Fund (ERCF), a mechanism established by the Conservative government in November 1995 and operated according to market principles of competitive bidding between authorities. As a condition of receiving money through the scheme, councils had to agree, and secure the agreement of its tenants, to transfer housing to Registered Social Landlords. The Labour government endorsed these rules, providing a record £248 million to the next round of ERCF funding in February 1998. Thereafter, ballots which led to tenants' approval for transfer were routinely referred to as 'successful', while councils were only able to 'win' funding by parading their own failures. The announcement of the February 1998 funding, for example, was accompanied by a list of 'winners' in the ERCF competition: 'This is one of St Helens' worst estates' being a typical example. By July, the results of third round ERCF bidding were known. The £248 million had been allocated to 15 local authorities covering 22,000 homes on 58 estates (DETR 1998e).

The further strand in New Labour's dealing with the public/private inter-face in housing thus revolves around its development of the previous adminis-tration's Private Finance Initiative (PFI). Chapter 8, dealing with privatisation and the National Health Service, has already set out some of the principles and practices which the previous administration introduced through the Private Finance Initiative. In opposition, the Labour Party had displayed a fondness for public/private partnerships in relation to capital programmes and some of this was translated into government. Before the end of 1997 a detailed document had been published (DETR 1997g) which committed £250 million in 1997/98 and a further £500 million in 1998/99 to public–private partnerships of a PFI kind. By June 1998 (DETR 1998b) a range of schemes had already been identi-fied, encompassing the whole range of public services, including the building of schools, hospitals and housing. Fifty-one PFI schemes were in operation in local government alone.

The enthusiasm of the new Government for private finance, competitive funding mechanisms and the celebration of transferring housing out of local authority control, illustrate some of the limitations of its willingness to substitute public effort and responsibility for private. This reservation extended to service provision by public bodies, as well as to questions of ownership. Compulsory Competitive Tendering (CCT) had been inherited from the Conservative era when, as earlier chapters have demonstrated, local government services had been progressively exposed to marketisation strategies. As a result, local author-ities were very often only able to provide services directly if the work involved had first gone out to tender and been won in open competition. By 1991, the system embraced a wide range of both manual and professional services. Labour fought the 1997 election with a manifesto commitment to replace CCT with a duty on local authorities to achieve Best Value in services provision. In practice, as ideas developed, it became clear that marketisation and competition were to remain as basic components of the Best Value. Indeed, the establishment of a Best Value Partnership Network was to be piloted in 1998/99 with the explicit remit of 'promoting use of the market to get better value for local authority in-house resources' (DETR 1998f).

Finally, in this section on people who rent their homes, it is worth noting another important element within Labour's developing policy, the proposals for dealing with 'nuisance neighbours' which had formed a prominent part of the Party's pre-election policy-making (see, for example, *Protecting Our Communities*, Labour Party 1997). These proposals found an immediate place in the first legislative programme of the incoming Government. The Crime and Disorder Bill provided for an Anti-Social Behaviour Order (ASBO) which allowed for the immediate arrest of any individual breaching its terms (DETR 1997h). By the time the Bill had become an Act of Parliament, the force of its social authoritarianism had become clearer. Anti-Social Behaviour Orders were to be available to the Court on the basis of a *civil* standard of proof – that is to say, on the balance of probabilities – where the word of a council officer would be sufficient to establish that such behaviour had taken place. In the event of an order being breached, however, a *criminal* offence would have taken place, punishable by a term of imprisonment of up to twelve months. The Act made ASBOs available for children as young as ten years old. In terms of the debate which occupies this book, the approach shows a willingness to use public measures to deal with circumstances where previously private remedies only would have applied. A paradox emerges here. On the one hand, policy development suggested a new willingness to extend the scope of public action. On the other, the effect of new public powers was to place additional responsibilities upon private individuals, with draconian consequences for them – in terms of losing accommodation and liberty – if they failed to comply. The social authoritarian agenda was a significant one for New Labour and, as later elements in this chapter and Chapter 10 will demonstrate, was to be influential in most social policy areas. In housing, the willingness to criminalise those who failed to meet new obligations – and thus privatising the consequences of social failure – suggested a key distinction in New Labour thinking. The benefits of a reinvigorated public policy were to be extended to those prepared to abide by the behavioural standards set down by the administration. For those unwilling or unable to do so, the result would be to be shut out of the newly-restricted circle of citizenship and to be left to bear the consequences for themselves.

Those who have no homes at all

It was, perhaps, in the area of homelessness which the new administration of May 1997 showed itself most willing to depart from the policies of its predecessors. As Chapter 4 suggested, the issue of homelessness had fallen into neglect during the Conservative years, with privatising policies designed either to remove the worst manifestations of a growing problem from public view or to reduce the entitlements to permanent housing which homeless people had previously been able to call upon. The approach of the incoming Government was very different. The Rough Sleepers Initiative which the previous administration had begun was given a new prominence with announcements of additional funding outside London in June, August, November and December 1997, extending provision to hitherto neglected areas such as Bath, Bournemouth, Cambridge and Chester. More significantly still, the spirit in which rough sleeping was to be addressed fell within a strategic approach to combating exclusion. The Social Exclusion Unit, set up by the Prime Minister in December 1997 and located within the Cabinet Office had, as one of its first priority areas, the development of a strategy to reduce rough sleeping to as low a level as possible. The resulting report was published in July 1998 (SEU 1998a). In terms of the focus of this book, the most significant element lies in the clear acceptance, in the Prime Ministerial Foreword, of public responsibility for addressing the issues raised. The spirit with which this responsibility was embraced marks a very clear distinction between the social privatisation of its predecessors and the new administration. As the Foreword ends, 'The most vulnerable should not be left simply to fall through the cracks in the system or have the odds so heavily stacked against them. This is a problem that has been with us too long and ruined too many lives. It is time to solve it.' The report was followed up by action in relation to young homeless people and, in September 1998, by a new Homeless Action Programme backed by £34 million over three years.

Some of the same urgency applied to Rough Sleepers was also evident in the government's approach to homelessness more generally. A consultation paper was issued on 22 May 1997, requiring responses to proposals to place new duties on local authorities in relation to homeless people by 20 June. As a result, the lessening of the obligations of local authorities towards homeless people contained in the 1996 Housing Act were overturned. The link between homelessness and the allocation of long-term social housing was restored, with homeless households placed again on the list of persons to be given reasonable preference in the allocation of social housing. Where local authorities discharged their obligation by assisting a homeless household to obtain private accommodation, a new requirement was added that authorities must be satisfied that the accommodation would be available to the household for at least two years (DETR 1997i).

Comprehensive spending review

One of the major landmarks of the new administration, across the whole of the social policy areas, came with the outcome of the Comprehensive Spending Review which brought to an end the self-imposed two-year period in which the new government had pledged itself to remain within the global spending levels inherited from its predecessor. The review promised £5 billion in extra spending on housing and regeneration projects over a three-year period. A New Deal for Regeneration and a revamped Single Regeneration Budget contributed further additional finance and focus upon what the government called 'intensive help to some of the country's most deprived neighbourhoods'. The outcome was hailed by the Chartered Institute of Housing as 'the first serious increase in housing resources for 10 years'. Once again, the scheme adopted the strategy of the previous Conservative administration in awarding the available finance through competitive bidding.

The New Deal for Regeneration was announced by the Prime Minister himself, speaking at Hackney in London, in a move which mirrored his decision to make the first major speech of his administration at a community centre on a run-down estate in Peckham. The New Deal demonstrated a series of strands in the new government's approach to public and private responsibilities. On the one hand, the scheme aimed to draw together a wide range of public bodies in a concerted effort to apply the benefits of determined public effort to some of the most concentrated areas of social difficulty. Long-term investment was promised, in order to overcome what the Social Exclusion Unit described as invariable failure of the repeated application of top-down, short-term solutions to structural causes of decline. Seventeen 'pathfinder' districts and eighteen special teams involving Whitehall departments, outside experts, community organisations and businesses were to be applied to finding new solutions.

Alongside this reinvigoration of public effort, however, the initiative contained a strong streak of New Labour morality in which regeneration was to be applied to the human as well as the physical stock of an area. Making the announcement of the £800 million deal, Mr Blair emphasised the 'high price of dependency' caused by poor neighbourhoods. The investment on offer, therefore, was to expect a return in the changed behaviour of people, as well as in the fabric of their surroundings.

The overall picture in relation to the private/public interface in housing under Labour is thus a mixed one. Undoubtedly, this was a Government where public spending and public responsibility were embraced to an extent unthinkable under its predecessor. In that process, a number of areas which had been ejected from the public ambit – in relation to homelessness, for example – were returned to the realm of collective responsibility. In other areas, however, market mechanisms were either moderated – as in the substitution of Best Value for CCT – or actively promoted, as in the case of the PFI and transfer of council housing. The Minister's distrust of ideology had been borne out in practice. Whether the new arrangements would all pass the 'doing what works' test is more open to question.

9.2 Social security

Labour came to office in May 1997 with an election promise to cut welfare bills. Perhaps more than in any other area, apart from law and order, the policy stance of the Party in relation to social security had undergone a transformation while in opposition. In office, some actions were to be defended on the same anti-ideological basis used by Housing Ministers. The decision to proceed with the privatisation of the Benefit Agency Medical Service, for example, was justified by Keith Bradley, the Minister responsible, on the basis that his was not a government of 'outdated ideology' or of 'dogmatic views' (DSS 1998a). In reality, however, the New Labour approach to social security was sharply ideological, rejecting much of the Party's own previous policy and freely adopting different approaches. Traditionally Labour, as the founding font of the welfare state, had been committed to the basic Beveridge principles of universal benefits, paid for through social insurance and progressive taxation. In the final period of opposition, however, and particularly under the leadership of Tony Blair, the Party had come to regard the social security system as part of the problem of welfare in Britain, rather than part of a solution. The extent to which this realignment implies a reassignment of responsibility between public and private, between the individual and the collective, forms the subject matter of this section.

In opposition

The effort to create social security policy which retained the support of Labour's own members while broadening the basis of its political appeal proved problematic from the outset. One of the main initiatives launched by John Smith, during his leadership of the Party, was the establishment of the *Commission on Social Justice* (Borrie 1994). This body, which drew its membership from beyond the Labour Party, provided a report which rejected the free market approaches of Thatcherism – which it characterised as 'deregulators Britain' – and the public ownership and redistributive policies of traditional Labourism – which it described as 'levellers Britain'. Instead it preferred 'investors Britain', a place where opportunity rather than simply money would be redistributed in favour of those in need. In the sound-bite of the day, the report suggested a system which would offer a 'hand up, not a hand out'. Social security was to be achieved by placing a new emphasis on the preparation of people for work and on a mixed economy of welfare, in which public and private solutions were both to play a part. The system would become 'a spring-board to success, not a safety net to cushion failure'.

By the time of the General Election, Labour's policy had formalised around the new ground. The argument presented suggested that social security represented the cost of failure, in which billions of pounds were spent to universal dissatisfaction. The system no longer gained the support of either those who paid for it or those who were paid by it, neither those who worked for it nor those who depended upon it. The challenge for the new administration was to find ways of spending less on mopping up the casualties of economic failure, and more on investing in the conditions of success. If expenditure on passive social security could be reduced, money could then be redirected to investment in the improvement of active services of health and education. Under Labour, policies emerged through which bills were to be reduced in two ways. Firstly, wherever possible, social security claimants were to be moved from welfare to work. Secondly, the methods of providing for sickness, old age and other contingencies were no longer to be regarded as solely the province of the state. A wider range of instruments, including the private sector, were to be employed. Through all these conclusions a linking theme was clear, as the Prime Minister made explicit in his first set-piece speech following the election victory: 'We have reached the limits of the public's willingness simply to fund an unreformed welfare state through ever higher taxes and spending' *[document 11]*. Moreover, whatever spending might prove possible would have to be organised on the basis of a new reciprocity in the relationship between the claimant and the system. Peter Mandleson and Roger Liddle (1996), in an influential pre-election publication, put it in sharp tones:

'It is not right that some people should collect the dole, live on the black economy, and then refuse to co-operate with society's efforts to reintegrate them into the labour market. It is dishonest and corrosive of our attempt to build a sense of mutual obligations in the community. In circumstances where new opportunity is being offered and refused, there should be no absolute entitlement to continued receipt of full social security benefits.'

In government

Measured against the high ambitions with which Labour entered office, the early record of the new Government suggested that welfare reform was to prove an even more contentious and difficult area than had been anticipated. Social security policy provided the greatest upheavals within a usually-pliant Parliamentary Labour Party while, politically, the first Prime Ministerial reshuffle of his cabinet saw the sacking of the Secretary of State and the resignation of the Minister for Welfare Reform, an outcome which Lloyd (1998: 33) described as 'an index of the fearsome difficulties of recasting a welfare system in a democracy'. In mid-term, the policy area remained one where great reforms were planned, but where action continued to be delayed, the promised radicalism more evident in potential than in action.

It cannot be an ambition of this chapter to trace in detail the day-to-day actions of New Labour in the social security field. A number of key policy trends, however, can be discerned which are directly relevant to the focus of this text. These themes are now explored, followed by a brief consideration of the application of such ideas in specific policy areas.

Making policy

The central ideas of the first period of New Labour social security policy-making were expressed by Ministers in a number of key-note speeches, delivered at symbolic events within the social welfare calendar. Two examples, occurring within a month of one another, must stand as symbolic of this wider intellectual effort – the Beveridge Memorial Lecture provided by the Minister for Welfare Reform, Frank Field, on 18 February 1998, and the speech of the Secretary of State, Harriet Harman, at the University of York Conference to mark the Centenary of Seebohm Rowntree's First Study of poverty in that city.

The Beveridge Memorial lecture (Field 1998) was Frank Field's final public platform, prior to the unveiling of the Green Paper on Welfare Reform, a document billed as setting out, in a seminal way, the translation of the Government's general intention in the welfare area into practical measures. He planned, he told his audience, to use the lecture to 'draw together the main themes' which were to underpin the Green Paper. Central to those themes was the diminution which Ministers claimed to have taken place in public support for the social security system since its post-war origins. That support, said Mr Field, had worn away 'in a remarkable way'. As a result, government was no longer regarded by the electorate as the natural or inevitable provider of welfare. More would need to be spent in the future, in order to provide for social security, but the proportion of that greater bill met through direct taxation would have to fall. A division of risk would have to be undertaken between those covered through collective provision organised by government and those 'which should sensibly be undertaken by people individually, or through other forms of collective cover'. In other words, the main pillar of welfare reform was to be a redistribution, not of money, but of responsibility, in which individuals would be expected to shoulder a greater proportion of the burden of providing for themselves.

The themes in the Beveridge lecture did not, of course, belong to Mr Field alone. From May 1997 onwards, the new Secretary of State, Harriet Harman, had placed greater emphasis upon the ways in which the Blair administration would differ from previous Labour governments rather than from its Conservative predecessors. Ministers consciously adopted some of the marketising language of the previous administration. 'Claimants' were out, and 'customers' were in (DSS 1997a). By contrast, 'rights' were no longer part of mainstream Labour vocabulary. Rather, from her very first public remarks, the new Secretary of State referred to welfare payments as 'state handouts' (DSS 1997b) which were costly to the taxpayer and undermining to the dignity of recipients. The system was to be reformed in order 'to reduce poverty and welfare dependency and promote work incentives' (DSS 1997c) and the use of private as well as public providers was explicitly to be included within that framework. A series of such themes was brought together in a keynote speech made at York (Harman 1998), one month after the Field Beveridge lecture and one week ahead of the Green Paper. The views of the Secretary of State were plain: a benefits-led strategy for assisting people in poverty was 'increasingly expensive' and served 'no good effect'. The 'real enemy' of equality was 'not just income distribution' but 'lack of education, skills, and the kind of practical support that enables people to get jobs'. In other words, the 'heart of Labour's strategy' was to be 'a reaffirmation that work for those who can is a fundamental responsibility of the citizen'.

In terms of the debates which form the focus of this book, these ministerial contributions identify some core beliefs which underpinned the New Labour approach to social security. Both Ministers were agreed that the division of responsibility between state and individual would have to be redrawn, with individual citizens accepting greater responsibility for securing their own incomes, both through work and through a greater contribution towards the costs of an income when sick, unemployed or old. Governments retained a responsibility for creating the conditions in which individuals were able to meet these obligations, either through education and skills acquisition or through the promotion of a mixed economy of insurance-based arrangements to cover periods when work was not possible. When the Green Paper on Welfare Reform was published in March 1998, the introduction by the Prime Minister re-employed a slogan which Labour had developed to characterise its welfare approach, 'we want to rebuild the system around work and security. Work for those who can; security for those who cannot.' Commenting on the document, Hills (1998: 28) notes the difference between this formulation and the 'security for all' basis of the post-war Beveridge system. As Hills suggests, 'it is hard to imagine that this is an accidental slip'.

149

Within these broad patterns, therefore, some additional debates were concealed which were less amenable to resolution. In the case of welfare-to-work policies, for example, where was the balance to be struck between encouragement and requirement? In the case of the market for welfare insurance, where was the line to be drawn between individual choice and compulsion? It was these tensions, rather than the headline themes which were to bring about the extinction of Labour's first social security ministry during the summer of 1998.

Frank Field left the Blair administration of his own volition, having been denied the post of Secretary of State for Social Security. In a series of briefings and counter-briefings which followed over the next few days, it soon became clear that his departure represented a defeat over a fundamental principle of social security policy: universality as against means-tested benefits. The Field blue-print for welfare reform included an emphasis upon private rather than public provision, but – as his earlier writings had long made clear – he favoured an element of compulsion in relation to individual welfare-planning which would have insisted, for example, upon all working citizens making provision for second-tier pensions. Only in this way, he argued, could a universal welfare system be maintained, and an income be provided for individuals which would be sufficient for survival without recourse to the moral-sapping measures of the means-test. On the other side, however, the Treasury were less convinced. Compulsory pension contributions would appear as a tax to those obliged to make them, and would leave the general revenue with a substantial bill in making provision for those whose work patterns or health condition would never allow for a personal pension to be built up in the way envisaged. The Treasury was in the grip of the means-testers, for whom a sharper distinction was to be drawn between the 'targeted' provision to be made for those unable to look after themselves, and the more interference-free responsibility of others to make their own arrangements. In his resignation speech to the House of Commons, Field reserved his greatest scorn for the notion that means-testing could provide the basis of a worthwhile social security system. It was responsible, he said, for 'the cancerous impact that much of welfare has on people's motivation, their actions and thereby their character'.

The fall of Harriet Harman was less the outcome of a sharpening ideological battle than the product of the unsteady course which, under her direction, had been chartered between the conflicting demands of policy making. The emphasis upon work, rather than welfare, had never adequately answered the question of job creation, or addressed the nature of employment on offer and its remuneration. As Fitzpatrick (1998) suggests, the policy concentrated upon the virtues of work, regardless of quality. In practice, the Government's policy was almost wholly supply-sided, emphasising the need for unemployed young people, single parents, disabled people and so on to better prepare themselves for employment. The demand side of the equation – where were the jobs to be found? – was treated as part of some Keynsian twilight, over which the Government had little or no control. Against that background, benefit cuts for lone parents and a creeping compulsion towards participation in New Deal-type schemes met with suspicion and outright rejection.

The replacement of the unhappy Harman/Field combination with Alistair Darling as Secretary of State moved an ultra-loyalist of the Blair project into the welfare reform arena. In a speech to the Institute of Public Policy Research in September 1998 *[document 13]* he began to outline the new emphasis which he intended to bring to the Ministry. Three aspects are especially worth noting. Firstly, the speech included a fresh enthusiasm for private sector provision: social security, said Mr Darling, 'isn't and shouldn't be a monopoly of the public sector. Far from it. . . . Where the post-war pioneers thought of state provision as an alternative to private provision, today we need a partnership between public and private sectors.' Secondly, the speech laid new emphasis upon the responsibilities, rather than the rights of citizens. In relation to child poverty, for example, the Minister chose to begin his consideration by emphasising the government's determination 'that parents face up to their responsibilities' by supporting their children through the education system. Finally, the Minister signalled a resolution of the debate between a universal or means-tested welfare system in favour of the latter. Claiming that the choice between 'means-testing' and a 'contributory' system represented a 'false dichotomy', the speech still made it clear, in unalloyed means-testing language, that 'state spending should be concentrated where it is needed most' and resources 'directed to the best possible effect'.

The policy direction set out in the Alistair Darling speech represents more than a change of emphasis or nuance. In the assessment of Will Hutton (writing in *The Observer* on 2 August 1998), the decision to pursue a means-testing rather than universalist strategy is one which 'defines high politics'. In arriving at this conclusion the government had turned its back on the radical strategy of a reinvented universalism, based on social insurance, which would have had social solidarity as its central aim through providing 'a rational response to life's hazards and a vital support system for every citizen necessarily confronted by the instability and inequity of capitalism'. In its place had come the triumph of a neo-conservative model, with an emphasis on keeping taxes down, in which individuals take their own chance, as best they may, and which regards the government's role as confined to securing reasonable education and training and providing other help only when it is demonstrably needed. Hall (1998: 12) suggests that New Labour's decision to adopt the means-testing route to welfare reform will include an inevitable propulsion towards private provision, for those able to afford it. The broader public interest in maintaining quality services for all will be weakened in the process, leaving those requiring state assistance propelled ever more towards the margins.

In terms of the concerns of this book, the choices which Hutton describes contain within them very different models of the relationship between public and private responsibility. The social insurance model is one in which the state undertakes final accountability for ensuring that all citizens have a common interest in collective as well as individual well-being. The neo-conservative model,

151

by contrast, regards individuals as essentially responsible for themselves, but only for themselves. The state's obligation is a residual one, picking up only those who cannot make provision through their own efforts, or through their own resources. Hutton's verdict summarises the outcome succinctly, in terms of the preoccupations of this book. As New Labour enters the middle period of its 1997 administration, 'the process of opting out and partial privatisation of the welfare system will accelerate'.

Applying social security principles

If these were some of the key ideas which guided the making of social security policy under New Labour, space allows only a brief exploration of a small number of instances where these ideas were translated into practical action. This section begins with a consideration of a range of Labour's policies upon those individuals for whom the system offered not 'opting-out' but deliberate ejection. It then turns to one specific area of policy development, that of pension reform.

Individuals and social authoritarianism

The conditional and contractual view of social security had been clearly set out by Tony Blair in his post-election Aylesbury estate speech. The Prime Minister *[document 11]* put it in this way: 'The basis of this modern civic society is an ethic of mutual responsibility or duty. It is something for something, a society where we play by the rules. You only take out if you put in. That's the bargain.' It is beyond the scope of this chapter to consider the single most important example of New Labour's social security bargain, the New Deal, other than to note its central role in transferring responsibility from the public sphere of welfare to the private sphere of work, in partial fulfilment of the New Labour mantra: 'Work for those who can; security for those who cannot.' An excellent discussion of the general issues inherent in the policy is to be found in Deacon (1997). At the Aylesbury estate, the Prime Minister promised an investment of £4 billion in the New Deal for young people, producing 'quality jobs' or 'full-time education and training, to provide the foundation for getting a job in the future'. In a departure from his Party's Election Manifesto, however, he also made it clear that, for those young people unwilling to play by these rules, 'there will be and should be no fifth option of an inactive life on benefit'.

The classification of young people into the 'willing' and 'unwilling' is emblematic of an older and deeper division in British welfare thinking and represents a recategorisation of the poor into those ingrained groupings of the deserving and the undeserving. New Labour's capacity for dividing the social world into those who are worthy of assistance and those who are in need of restraint is a sharp one, and marks one of the major boundaries between this and earlier Labour governments. Fitzpatrick (1998: 18), in discussing the communitarian philosophy to which New Labour laid claim, suggests that policy making has been derived from a version of that agenda which is 'conformist and prescriptivist in its adherence to a moralistic conservatism'.

Finer Jones (1997: 169) provides a useful analysis of these changes in terms of the stakeholding vocabulary which Labour politicians, especially when in opposition, had appropriated. She suggests that stakeholdership aimed to replace the Thatcherite onslaught on welfare culture with 'a culture of incentives and disincentives capable of shaping behaviour in ways to benefit each and everyone together'. The hidden message within stakeholding, however, is that, as in market relationships, this structure of incentives produces both 'winners and losers, not just winners'. Governments are responsible for creating the conditions in which each citizen is able to receive a fair chance of making something of her or his life. The responsibility for taking that chance lies with the individual. Those who do not will have demonstrated their lack of suitability for further state investment. Three subdivisions of individuals may be found among this group of non-deservers, each of which has relevance to the development of Labour's social security policy. The first category are those whom Finer Jones calls the non-stakeholders. These are the economic migrants and suspect asylum seekers of Fortress Europe. The second are the passive resisters of stakeholding – those, for example, who fail to seek work actively enough to satisfy the new enforcers of the New Deal or Job Seekers Allowance. Thirdly, there are the anti-stakeholders, the cheats and frauds of the benefit system.

As far as non-stakeholders are concerned, Labour's approach has little by which it can easily be distinguished from that of its predecessors. Labour's record on immigration and asylum issues has long been one in which a tension emerges between liberal impulses and authoritarian actions. The metamorphosis to 'New' Labour diluted the former while strengthening the latter. Labour was to be as 'tough' on 'bogus' asylum seekers as any other deviant group. In office, while the language of 'fairness' once again entered the vocabulary, action remained predicated upon fear and suspicion. Prodded along by successive scare stories – Romanian gypsies, Kosovan refugees – the policy has produced further erosions of the very limited social and civil rights bequeathed by the previous administration.

The second group, the passive resisters, represents the greatest challenge for New Labour, both numerically and ideologically. The 'no fifth option' applied to young people and the New Deal has already been noted above. As the administration became more established, the compulsion with which such responsibilities were to be awoken and the consequences where that did not occur, were extended to groups against whom the previous administration had not moved with such determination. The New Deal for Lone Parents, for example, had been introduced with an explicit promise of its voluntary nature. The scheme was barely a year old, however, before the rules were altered to place new obligations to attend for interview, with greater penalties for those who failed to do so. The Queen's Speech of November 1998, which announced the legislative programme for the central period of the administration, carried this still further. A single gateway to the benefit system for those of working age was proposed – the Orwellian-sounding Single Work-Focused Gateway – in which compulsory participation would be required, with financial consequences for those refusing such assistance. The Welfare Reform Bill published early in 1999 formalised the Single Work-Focused Gateway to benefit (DSS 1999a), making 'discussion of a claimant's capacity for work a precondition for the receipt of benefits' and, in the case of JSA claimants, obliging them to follow further compulsory courses of action, in order for a claim to benefit to be sustained (DSS 1999b). In the terms suggested here, compulsion in enforcing responsibility had become part of the wider social authoritarian agenda upon which the administration was willing to rely.

As to the third group, the new administration's approach to social security fraud bordered on the obsessional. For Frank Field (DSS 1997d) 'the fight against fraud is an expression of responsible citizenship'. Harriet Harman (DSS 1998b) announced a new Benefit Fraud Inspectorate as 'welfare reform in action'. A fraud auction appeared to set in among Ministers, with each competing to produce the highest figure of claimant corruption. In March 1988 the Green Paper on Welfare Reform had suggested a probable level of fraud within the system of £4 billion each year. By July, a further DSS document, *Beating Fraud is Everyone's Business*, had suggested a figure of £7 billion. Even the briefest consideration of the way in which such sums were derived suggests how the public presentation of fraud had come to be driven by dogma rather than fact. The £7 billion figure had been arrived at by adding together £2 billion of confirmed fraud, £3 billion where the Department possessed 'strong suspicion' and £2 billion where, in the Ministry's own definition, 'the balance of probabilities is not met, nor is there usually enough evidence for a claim to be adjusted'.

Rowlingson *et al.* (1997) show that fraud explains only a very small portion of the benefits bill. Walker and Park (1998: 29), drawing on this and other evidence, rightly conclude that New Labour's policy in this area is thus 'rooted in ideology rather than evidence'. Indeed, New Labour's actions in this area are consistent with Le Grand's (1997) more general characterisation of a shift in policy-makers' beliefs about human motivation and behaviour in social welfare, in which the knights (public service workers) and pawns (welfare benefit recipients) of the Fabian welfare state have been replaced by a combined view of both as potential, if not actual, knaves. The ideology which informs the fraud policy represents a particular extension of this general administration approach in the social security area. For New Labour, too many people had come to depend on benefit. That dependency was often unnecessary and consisted of large numbers of people who were on welfare whereas they should be in work. Fraud emerges from the speeches of Ministers as an extension of this line of reasoning. Whole swathes of claimants, it could be implied, were fraudulently engaged in claiming benefits when they could have been taking care of themselves. On the basis of that blurred distinction, administrative penalties could be applied, in the place of the criminal law. The implementation of the Conservative government's Fraud Act 1997 fell to the new administration. It did so with alacrity, including the powers which the Act contained to allow benefit agency staff to impose administrative penalties instead of prosecution for fraud, 'where the overpayment is small and the nature of the fraud is minor' (DSS 1998c). The practical implementation of a socially authoritarian agenda thus included an additional twist to the moving boundary of public and private responsibility. As welfare rights advisers and others pointed out, vulnerable claimants, without due process of law and under the threat of prosecution, would be laid open to agreeing to penalties for offences which had never taken place. Simultaneously, the powers of the state had been increased while the operation and consequences of that increased power had been transferred out of the public sphere.

Policies in action: pension reform

The early history of New Labour's administration of social security suggests a government whose willingness to disengage from public responsibility outran that of its supporters. The effect was clearly apparent in the progress of pension reform, one of the great policy challenges facing the New Labour administration and one which was inherently controversial. While in opposition, the disputes which followed the Borrie Report (1994) centred most fiercely around pensions, with the former Cabinet Minister, and Secretary of State for Social Security, Barbara Castle, joining the doyen of social scientists, Peter Townsend, to publish a pamphlet setting out the case for universal pensions, funded through social insurance and up-rated in line with rising earnings, rather than prices. The Party's shadow Minister, Harriet Harman, disagreed. She suggested a new arrangement, in which the state pension would occupy a relatively residual position, bolstered by a new layer of second – or 'stakeholder' – pensions, for which the individual would be obliged to take responsibility.

The Party Manifesto sought a way out of this disagreement by promising a review of the long-term arrangements for pension provision. In government a Pension Provision Group was quickly established. Among its terms of reference was an explicit remit to 'establish the right balance between the public and private sectors' (DSS 1997e). The group reported in June 1998, but the government's response was delayed by ministerial changes and policy disagreements, until the publication of its pensions Green Paper *A New Contract for Welfare: Partnership in Pension* (DSS 1998d) in December 1998. By that time a number of policy initiatives had already developed, in response to a series of reports which identified the problems of poorest pensions (see, for example, Legard *et al.* 1998). These included a guaranteed minimum income of £75 for single pensioners from April 1999, the re-introduction of free eye tests for pensioners, consolidation of new Winter Fuel Payments and additional travel concessions on public transport (DSS 1998e). Additional expenditure of some £2.5 billion was to be devoted to these purposes.

The initiatives aimed at poorest pensioners, however, masked a deeper debate taking place within government concerning the incomes of future generations of people in retirement. The December 1998 Green Paper proposed a new 'Insurance Contract' through which future arrangements would be made.

Two central decisions shaped the policy suggestions contained within the Contract. Firstly, the government rejected the Castle/Townsend suggestion that the state should re-assume responsibility for providing a decent income in retirement by, for example, raising the basic state pension in line with earnings. The Paper rejected this universalist approach in favour of 'focusing extra state support on those who need it most'. Secondly, the government rejected the notion of compulsory contributions to second-tier pensions, an idea which had been most closely associated with the departed Minister, Frank Field. The Welfare Reform Green Paper published by Mr Field in March 1998 placed compulsion firmly on the agenda. As suggested earlier, the December Pensions Green Paper rejected the idea on the grounds that the government did not now 'believe we should force people to save more or that we need to'. In its place, the document proposed new state-supported and provided arrangements for low earners and non-earners, together with private sector pensions for those in middle and higher earning brackets. 'Stakeholder pensions', brought into being by public–private partnerships, were, said the document, 'at the heart of our reforms'.

In terms of the concerns of this book, pension reform illustrates a number of essential elements within New Labour's formulation of public and private responsibility in the social security area. The December 1998 Green Paper includes a straightforward repudiation of the Beveridge notion of universal benefits, financed through social insurance contributions. The basic state pension was to remain, but would not provide the vehicle for mainstream provision in the future. In its place, individuals would be expected to take a much larger share of responsibility for providing for themselves in old age. The role of the government would be three-fold. For those able to look after themselves, the government would retain the responsibility for fostering and regulating private provision and providing incentives for individuals to bring themselves within private arrangements. For those in low-paid or irregular employment, the government proposed Second State Pensions, sufficient to raise their incomes in retirement above the means-tested limit. For the remainder, the basic state pension would continue, on a means-tested basis, to be made up to a guaranteed income level.

Whiteside (1998: 215) identifies a series of essential continuities between the agendas of 'New' Labour and the previous administration. Welfare reforms, he suggested, are 'still promising to separate the purchase of welfare from its provision, to involve consumer choice, to use central regulation of private agencies (rather than an extension of the public sector) as the main route to welfare reform'. Fitzpatrick (1998: 25) places these continuities in the wider context of changing public and private responsibilities. The purpose of social policy, at the end of the 1990s, has become, he suggests, 'less to fit institutions to individuals, but to fit individuals to institutions. If social legitimacy can no longer be ensured by the collective guarantee of security for all then it must derive from the deliberate lowering of individuals' expectations so that they correspond to the requirements of a supervisory, fee-paying state.'

9.3 Education

Labour entered the 1997 General Election with education as one of its foremost policy areas. The new Prime Minister had famously summed up the Party's priorities as, 'education, education, education'. Once in government, the new Secretary of State for Education and Employment, David Blunkett,[1] moved quickly to reinforce this message, declaring that, 'no Government Department's work is more important' (DFEE 1997a). In the competition for places in Labour's first legislative programme for nearly twenty years, education emerged with two Bills. The first set out to redeem a specific election pledge to reduce primary school class sizes for five-, six- and seven-year-olds to 30 by using money freed up through the abolition of the Assisted Places Scheme. The second set out the government's approach to raising educational standards through new measures to tackle under-achievement in schools; introducing base-line assessment of children, ending the grant-maintained schools programme and amending the framework for local management of schools.

This chapter cannot aim to provide a comprehensive account of the education policies of New Labour in office.[2] Not even all those elements which include significant realignments of the public–private interface can be discussed at length. Rather, my aim is to identify and discuss briefly a number of policy areas where the new administration's approach can be clearly distinguished from that of its predecessor, before turning to policies which showed greater continuities with its marketising and privatising inheritance.

Doing things differently?

During the Conservative years, the boundary between private and public in education, as Chapter 5 suggested, had been shifted towards private responsibility across a broad range of policy areas. Labour in office demonstrated a fresh belief in the power of government action to bring about social improvement and, in some areas at least, a scepticism about market rather than planning mechanisms in education. In this latter area, the new administration made

[1] To a greater extent than other social policy areas the information in this section refers specifically to developments in England. Scotland, of course, has a distinct and separate education system. Responsibility for education in Wales lies with the Welsh Office and, after May 1999, with the National Assembly for Wales. In the run-up to Assembly elections, Welsh Office ministers pursued an increasingly independent line in relation to education, mapping out a distinctive policy approach which did not share to the same degree the enthusiasms for inspection, testing, managerialism and marketisation which were characteristic of their English equivalents.

[2] In particular it does not deal at all with questions of Higher Education, including the extension of loans in place of grants and the introduction of tuition fees for students. In the terms of this book, both developments clearly belong to the privatising trend in social policy, in which responsibilities previously undertaken by the state are transferred to individuals.

Nor does it deal with the implementation, by the Labour government, of the previous administration's plans for the sale of student loan debt, a programme described by the Minister responsible as 'further evidence of our commitment to develop a wide range of public–private partnerships which transfer risk to the private sector' – a summary which might have been applied to a wide range of privatising policies during the 1980s and early 1990s (DFEE 1998a).

an early announcement of its intention to abolish the nursery voucher scheme, substituting 'partnership and co-operation' for 'damaging competition between providers' (DFEE 1997b). Authorities were invited to submit Early Years Development Plans through which four-year-olds might be guaranteed access to free education places. Significantly, when these plans were submitted early in 1998, the only ones which the Department required to be resubmitted were those where the government required 'a greater emphasis on working with voluntary and private providers' (DFEE 1998b). More generally, an ambitious programme of homework clubs and summer schools for children in more deprived areas saw £200 million from the National Lottery New Opportunities Fund devoted to setting up a national network of 8,000 homework clubs by 2001 (DFEE 1997c) and over 600 summer schools catering for over 18,000 children operating during the summer of 1998 (DFEE 1998c).

The new government also showed its willingness to apply the powers of intervention in addressing the social consequences of market operation in education. The Social Exclusion Unit produced, as its first major report, an investigation of school exclusion and truancy (SEU 1998b). The Department for Education and Employment responded with a commitment to reduce existing figures by a third by the year 2002 and provided £22 million to tackle the problem in 1997. As figures published in 1998 showed that the number of pupils permanently excluded had continued to rise in the last full year of Conservative administration (DFEE 1998d) – including a 21 per cent rise in the number of pupils excluded from special education – the government announced a more far-reaching £500 million programme to support action to reduce truancy and exclusion over a three-year period (DFEE 1998e). The Department also moved to counter one of the market advantages which some schools had hoped to secure through excluding pupils for the purposes of examination league tables. Such efforts, said the Minister, were an 'abuse of the system [which] . . . damages the children concerned and deceives parents and the public' (DFEE 1998f). Specifically acknowledging the impact of school marketisation upon the level of exclusions, the Social Exclusion Unit (SEU) report suggested, 'some feel the problem is that schools have been under such pressure to meet demanding academic standards and compete with each other, that excluding borderline cases could seem more attractive; performance tables have often been blamed for this'.

The attack of truancy and school exclusion, however, was not confined to altering the structural factors which had brought about the rise. The social authoritarianism identified in housing policy occurred again in relation to education. Truancy, for example, was the product of lax parenting on the one hand and the absence of sufficient enforcement activity by schools and local authorities on the other. The social authoritarianism. The boundary between private and public in social matters was realigned to allow for greater public intrusion into areas which had, hitherto, been a matter of private decision making. The homework clubs noted above, for example, came equipped with national guidelines, 'so that schools, parents and pupils realise the importance of homework in raising standards'. Issuing details of government-expected norms in homework – ten minutes on reading, ten minutes on 'other home activities' for infant reception children for example – the Secretary of State bemoaned research evidence that 43 per cent of all 10-year-olds had no regular homework, while over half spend three or more hours a night watching television (DFEE 1998g). One of his junior Ministers, in the meantime, had published information about new home–school contracts in which parents were to be obliged to sign a document including expectations about the standard of education, the ethos of the school, regular and punctual attendance, discipline and homework obligations (DFEE 1997d). Addressing a conference on parenting in his home city of Sheffield, the Secretary of State declared the government's policy to be one of being 'both tough and tender' towards parents, setting a framework within which 'intolerable behaviour' would not be accepted. Parents were not to be allowed an abdication of their responsibilities – 'all too often because parents claim not to have the time, because they have dis-engaged from their children's education'. He repeated a central theme of education policy – quite unlike that in the field of health, for example – that lack of progress in education was the product of 'poverty of expectation and dedication, and not so much the poverty of income' (DFEE 1998h).

The market framework

If there were education policy areas in which New Labour set about developing a distinctive agenda, the more striking characteristic of its early efforts in this field appeared in the continuities which occurred between its approach and the market framework which its predecessors had developed over almost ten years. Over that period the Party had already accommodated itself to some of these changes, as its early record in government indicated. One of the earlier amendments to traditional Labour policy in education had come, for example, with the acceptance of the Conservative reforms in relation to delegation of budgets to school level. Most often, however, that acceptance had been accompanied by a Labour reaffirmation of the role of local education authorities as supplier of services which were needed on a cross-school basis, such as school meals, education psychology services, grounds maintenance and so on. The administration in government, however, moved to introduce a new scheme for 100 per cent delegation of budgets, in which almost all services would be provided by schools making their own arrangements, or purchasing elements back from the local education authority (DFEE 1998i). The reforms gave all state schools the same degree of financial independence that was available to grant-maintained schools. The scheme was criticised for undermining economies of scale, offering schools recycled money rather than any new money, and for creating new bureaucracy in terms of contracting arrangements between schools and LEAs. In terms of the central debates of this book, the move suggested that Labour's education policy shared many of the characteristics of its neo-liberal predecessors – distrust of local education authorities and a preference for the market to regulate the supply and demand of basic school services. Placing money in the hands of consumers of such services (schools) rather than providers (local education authorities) would, said the new Ministers in language which could have been adopted at any time since 1988, create choice and drive up standards *[document 12]*. Yet, faced with evidence of real increases in the number of appeals from parents unable to obtain a place at their school of choice, on the one hand, and growing numbers of surplus places on the other, the government relied upon a reassertion of market mechanisms: 'The supply of and demand for places must be brought more closely into balance so that parental preference can be maximised' (DFEE 1998j).

A second area in which New Labour's enthusiasm for the marketising agenda appeared to exceed even that of its predecessors lay in the emphasis it placed upon regimes of testing children as the means of driving up standards. Ministers repeatedly emphasised traditional, conservative notions of learning and the curriculum, in which 'a sharper focus on the three Rs' would be a priority' (DFEE 1997e). English teaching was to include grammar, spelling and punctuation, and mathematics was to focus on 'young people getting to grips with their tables and doing calculations in their heads rather than by pushing the buttons of a calculator' (DFEE 1997f).

Less than two weeks after taking office, new targets for achievement in national testing had been announced and a tone had been set for official pronouncements in education which was to remain characteristic of the government's policy in this area. The new targets were 'tough' and set by an administration which 'meant business' (DFEE 1997f). The new testing regime was to be 'tough' as well (DFEE 1997g). The purpose of such policies rested upon the essential need to provide market signals to parents in choosing schools for their children. The introduction of baseline testing for children entering infant school, introduced in September 1998 (DFEE 1998k), and the reduction of infant class sizes to 30 were both predicated upon the need to produce an enhancement of parental preference (DFEE 1997h). The outcomes of school testing were to be published, albeit in a new value-added format, because, Ministers said, 'Performance tables help focus debate on standards. Parents need the tables to inform their decisions about their children's future' (DFEE 1997i). The government was 'committed to providing the maximum amount of information to parents and pupils about school standards and ensuring that schools and LEAs use the information to help improve standards' (DFEE 1998l).

The determination of the privatisers to attack the privileges of producers of social welfare services and enthrone the consumer as king thus found fresh enthusiasts in Labour's educational team. Mr Blunkett freely adopted the language of neo-liberal orthodoxy when providing the annual lecture of the Technology Colleges Trust: 'We must move from an education system which caters for the producers to one which puts the needs of the consumers – pupils and their parents – at the heart of its approach' (DFEE 1997j) *[document 12]*. Within the first six weeks of the new administration, attacks had been mounted on a range of producer interests, including failing schools (7 May), failing teachers

(28 May) and failing local authorities (12 June). A language of aggressive machismo was again to the fore. There were to be 'tough new measures on failing schools' (DFEE 1997k) and a 'crackdown on failing teachers' (DFEE 1997l). Schools' Minister Steven Byres took the opportunity of an early debate on the new White Paper, *Excellence in Schools*, to call for incompetent teachers to 'be sacked within weeks'. There was, said the same Minister, to be 'zero tolerance' of delays in such procedures, including those arising from sickness (DFEE 1997m). The opposite side of this coin was to be found in the early announcement of 'superteachers' (DFEE 1997n) and a new grade of Advanced Skills Teacher (ASTs) capable of being paid up to £40,000 a year. The roots of ASTs were recognisably to be found in the performance-related pay policies of the previous Conservative administrations, where the New Right had regarded national pay arrangements as one of the major stumbling blocks in creating a free market in the supply and demand of labour. ASTs were to be employed on a different contractual basis, without the protection of working time limits applied to ordinary classroom teachers. Their annual pay progression would also be based not on an incremental scale but be subject to yearly performance reviews on the basis of agreed performance criteria. In 1999, this payment-by-results approach was extended to whole schools. The Prime Minister and the Education Secretary together announced an annual fund of £60 million 'to reward staff at schools which show excellent performance or significantly improve' (DFEE 1999a). The liberalising of the market, at both the hiring and firing ends, was thus more rapidly and far-reachingly undertaken under Labour than by its predecessors.

As well as tackling schools and teachers, New Labour turned its attention to local education authorities, declaring that in so far as they failed to comply with the new standards regime, 'they are part of the problem', rather than its solution (DFEE 1997o). The *School Standards and Framework Bill*, published in December 1997, duly included powers for central government to intervene in 'failing' local education authorities and to take-over their powers. The *School Standards Bill* in 1998 introduced five yearly inspections of LEAs by the Inspectorate OFSTED (DFEE 1998l). 'Tough New Targets' in literacy tests were set for local authorities, accompanied by a standard mantra of New Labour education policy makers: 'We want no excuses for failure. Many LEAs are in deprived areas, but poverty is no excuse for under-achievement' (DFEE 1998m). Early in 1999 the policy was taken a step further when the Education Secretary announced that the Department would advertise for contractors to take-over the key functions of failing LEAs (DFEE 1999b). Applications from not-for-profit and private service providers were explicitly invited, in what was widely identified as a further erosion of state responsibility in education.

The new government's emphasis upon 'standards, standards, standards' stood in deliberate contrast to the traditional Labour Party concerns with the structures of education provision. The new approach combined an attack upon the importance of structural reforms – particularly those of the comprehensive sort – with a range of structural changes of its own which emphasised the marketising virtues of diversity and choice. A series of initiatives aimed to provide variety in educational provision, most often involving a deliberate infusion of private sector interests. Within the first month of taking office, the Department agreed a grant-maintained application from a 118-pupil school for 4–9-year-olds (DFEE 1997p). Traditional Labour hostility towards private education was dismissed by the new Ministers as 'old prejudice' which needed to be buried (DFEE 1997q). 'Ours', declared Stephen Byres to the annual conference of the Girls School Association, 'is a modern, forward-looking government' which rejected 'dogma' in favour of an appreciation of the 'vital role which the independent sector plays within our education system'. A £1 million grant followed in October 1998 'to foster links with independent schools' (DFEE 1998n). The first comprehensive school teacher to address a conference of heads of private schools, the School Standards Minister Estelle Morris comforted delegates with an assurance that they were safe in Labour's hands. As she told reporters afterwards, 'There will always be people who choose to send children to these schools. They will always have that right under a Labour government' (*The Guardian* 8.10.98).

Within the state sector, the setting up of Education Action Zones (EAZs), designed to raise standards in struggling areas, were to be formed around a hierarchy of 'business, parents and local education authorities' (DFEE 1998o). Zones were to have market freedom to set different salary levels, to employ 'advanced skills teachers' and to change the emphasis of the National Curriculum, 'to focus more on literacy and numeracy standards'. Application to form an EAZ depended upon raising £250,000 from business and other local sponsorship. An accelerated programme of zone creation, and an increase in government funding from £250,000 to £750,000 for each zone was announced in April 1998 (DFEE 1998p). Hailing the passage of the *Schools Standards and Framework* Bill into law in July 1998, the Secretary of State singled out the EAZs as, 'a revolutionary and innovative partnership between businesses, parents, schools and Local Education Authorities to boost standards . . . [they] . . . will pump £75 million in three years into 25 areas facing real educational challenges' (DFEE 1998q). To others, the zones amounted to privatisation by the back door, drawing together a combination of private finance, the prioritising of business influence over public authorities and managerialist techniques which had all the hallmarks of neo-liberalism.

On an even larger scale, and with even more enthusiasm, the new administration took over and expanded the specialist schools programme of its predecessors. The programme had been launched in September 1993, beginning with the City Technology Colleges programme and had been extended in November 1994 to include modern foreign languages and then, in June 1996, to Sport and the Arts. The terms in which new Ministers embraced the initiative were recognisably those of the market. Such schools were 'popular with schools, parents and sponsors alike' (DFEE 1997r). Competition to achieve specialist status was 'intense' and depended upon each school raising £100,000 in private sector sponsorship to help improve the school's facilities in the specialist areas. Successful application would then release a further £100,000 in extra capital funding from the Department, together with extra annual funding for three years of £100 per pupil per annum. Once again, the case for the specialist schools programme was set out by Ministers in terms which emphasised the break with traditional Labour thinking and the embrace which had been extended to the policies of its privatising predecessors. David Blunkett's lecture to the Technology Colleges Trust (DFEE 1997j) *[document 12]* placed particular emphasis upon the initiative as a symbol of New Labour's thinking in education: 'Specialist schools are at the heart of my vision – and that of the new Government – of an education system where education caters for the individual strengths of children rather than assuming a bland sameness for all.'

Within the Labour Party, the greatest critic of its new education policy, former Deputy Leader Roy Hattersley, described Mr Blunkett's approach in this way: 'He has gone out of his way to offend all the principles – perhaps he now calls them prejudices – that have sustained party policy on schools.' He dismissed the insistence that standards were more important than structures in this way:

'The intellectual inadequacy of the argument – that how schools are organised has no effect on their results – is less important than its ideological implications. It is a denial of the basic socialist belief that the disadvantaged are often more the victims of society, than the product of their personal shortcomings.'

By the end of October 1998 the programme was further expanded. Now the 'flagship specialist schools programme' was to be expanded to 500 by 2002, making 'one in seven secondary schools a specialist school' (DFEE 1998r). Alongside it had been grafted a further 'Beacon School' initiative in which schools receiving especially good inspection reports were invited to bid for a share of a further £1.8 million (DFEE 1998s) in order to provide 'centres of excellence' for those around them. As many as 100 such schools were planned, each receiving up to £50,000 'to enable them to share the secrets of their success with others' (DFEE 1998t). The initiatives were further integrated in 1998 when it was announced that, in future, preference would be given to applications for specialist status from schools within EAZs (DFEE 1998u).

The justification for the 'diversity' provided by specialist and beacon schools was identified by Ministers as 'clear evidence that specialist schools do better than other comprehensives – 17 out of the 100 most improved secondary schools in the 1997 performance tables are specialist schools' (DFEE 1998v).

To those outside the government such conclusions were unsurprising. As Taylor-Gooby (1998) suggested, 'Shifts to "specialisation" or "choice" will undoubtedly be popular with the groups who make the most noise. But they will damage average levels of achievement by reducing educational attainment amongst those groups who have most to gain from schooling.' In other words, specialist schools and associated changes have the effect of privileging the chances of those who are already most advantaged. The creation of diversity and choice operates, as neo-liberals would expect, to allow the most powerful market actors

163

to obtain the best results for themselves. In the terms of such an explanation, the fact that specialist schools turn out to do well in examination league tables is less a reflection of their intrinsic merits than of their success in attracting pupils who would have done well in any other educational context. In practice, specialisation becomes simply a form of selection and one in which the distinction between aptitude and ability becomes indistinguishable. The result for those who lie outside the new circles of achievement, sponsorship and financial benefit is to struggle against renewed odds to provide a worthwhile education to children who remain behind.

Private Finance Initiative

Labour's use of the Conservative Private Finance Initiative has been explored earlier in this chapter in relation to housing, and space prevents a detailed account of its application in the field of education. The positive belief in the possibility of public action and public spending was not absent from the capital spending programmes of New Labour's education policy, but the additional benefits which were thought to be obtainable through private investment were a consistent theme in policy making. From the outset, David Blunkett identified public and private partnerships as the key to capital investment in school buildings (DFEE 1997s), with an emphasis upon the need for local authorities to find ways of making such partnerships more 'attractive to the private sector'. The first budget of the Labour government provided an additional £2 billion for schools, including £1.3 billion from the windfall tax to be spent on school repairs (DFEE 1997t). The Comprehensive Spending Review of July 1998 produced an additional headline figure of £19 billion for education, representing in real terms an average 3.4 per cent annual increase for English local authorities (DFEE 1998q).

Under Labour, the first school to be built through the PFI was instituted in Dorset (DFEE 1997u) on the basis that 'the PFI solution offers a practical means of completely rebuilding the school, at a lower cost than the traditional public sector route'. This success, and a further nine such projects, was celebrated by the Minister in a speech to the privatisation think-tank, the Adam Smith Institute, in which he 'welcomed the dramatic progress in public private partnerships in education' (DFEE 1998w).

The themes which thus emerge in relation to housing, social security and education are those already familiar from earlier chapters of this book. Determining the division of responsibility between state and individual, between public and private underpins the range of specific policies recounted here. The next chapter now turns to a pair of policy areas, social services and health, where the notion of reciprocity, both between individuals and between individuals and the state, has been particularly influential in the shaping of these relations.

Chapter 10

SOCIAL SERVICES AND HEALTH POLICIES AFTER 1997

10.1 Social services

When New Labour came to power in May 1997, its relatively slender manifesto had less to say in relation to social services than most other social policy areas. Even those commitments which had been entered into – to set up a Social Care Council and to institute independent regulation of residential and domiciliary care – were modest in comparison to the scale of its ambitions elsewhere. The early months of administration illustrated the contrast, within the same Ministry, between Labour's approach to health service reform and its attitude towards the personal social services. In health, Ministers were very swiftly into action, amending previous policy and proposing new initiatives of their own. In social services, the stance was primarily reactive, responding to crises in child care and further scandals in mental health, rather than seizing the initiative with any new or high-profile developments. Nevertheless, as the government settled into office, a number of strands within the social services came to receive more concentrated attention and to suggest the approach which Ministers would take in relation to the fundamental issue addressed in this text – the division of responsibility between the private spheres of family, individual and entrepreneurial initiative on the one hand and the acceptance of public responsibility – through funding and service delivery – on the other. The discussion which follows begins by looking at the nature and scale of social service expenditure inherited by the 1997 administration, before considering briefly its developing approach to children's services and the provision of care in the community. This section ends with a review of the most important social services initiative of the first two years of Labour in office, the White Paper, *Modernising Social Services [document 10b]* published in November 1998.

Costs

As Chapter 1 and Chapter 7 suggested, the personal social services were both relatively late in their development as a major public responsibility, and remained characterised by a mixed economy of public, voluntary and private provision throughout the post-1945 period. The transfer of responsibilities for care in the community to local authorities in 1993, however, led to a rise in overall public spending in this area. By 1996/97, for example, expenditure per head of the population in England on social services ran at an annual average of £189 and, over ten years, had risen by 89 per cent in real terms. From an expenditure of £9.3 billion in 1996/97, over £1 billion was now recouped in fees and charges from users (DoH 1998a). Within this general pattern, considerable variation was apparent between local authorities of apparently similar characteristics. Key statistics from the Department of Health (DoH 1998b) showed, for example, that the £189 per capita figure disguised a variation between local authorities of £95 at the lowest to £420 at the highest. Within that figure, gross weekly expenditure on residential care in local authority staffed homes for older people varied from £125 to over £750 per supported resident; gross expenditure per hour of home help/care in 1997/98 ranged between £5 and £30 and the percentage of social services departmental gross current expenditure recouped through fees and charges varied between 1 and 30 per cent.

Encompassed within the overall expenditure on social services were shifting patterns of responsibility between public and private forms of provision. While the majority of home care services were still provided directly by local authorities, the growth of independent providers had been rapid and substantial. In 1993 less than 5 per cent of contact hours had been drawn from the private sector. By 1996 this had risen to 36 per cent. Day care places were also shifting in the same direction. In a single year, between 1995 and 1996, the proportion of places provided by the private sector rose from 79 to 82 per cent (Personal Social Services Research Unit, 1997). Yet the trend towards concentration of growing services upon a shrinking number of individuals also continued. In domiciliary services, the number of contact hours increased by some 50 per cent between 1993 and 1997, while the number of households receiving services decreased by 7 per cent.

Children

The emphasis upon private provision during the 1980s and 1990s was felt in all social service sectors. Statistics showing the numbers and types of children's homes in England for the year to 31 March 1997, for example, demonstrate that privately registered homes represented the second largest group of providers (DoH 1998c). During that year, the Government responded reactively to the aftermath of a series of scandals in the child care field. In October 1997 the Social Services Inspectorate reported on the failure of Cambridgeshire County Council social services department to improve its performance in the wake of the death of Rikki Neave, a child who had been in the care of the authority. The report was met by stern words – 'those who persistently fail the vulnerable have no place in public life or the public service' – and threats of government intervention (DoH 1997a). November 1997 saw the publication of the Utting Report into safeguards for children living away from home (Utting 1997). The report had been commissioned in 1996 by the previous administration, in response to allegations of child abuse in residential care, dating back to the 1970s.

Among a series of conclusions, the report urged rapid action on the regulation of small, unregistered children's homes and identified children placed in private foster arrangements as extremely vulnerable and at considerable risk of abuse. At this stage, ministerial response concentrated upon forthcoming plans, rather than immediate change. Action was promised in relation to improved regulation and a future programme of 'policy and management changes to deliver the safer environment that children living away from home are entitled to' (DoH 1997b).

At the same time, in relation both to children and mental health services, the attacks upon community-based services had produced a creeping compulsion, in which use of the more formal and interventive powers of authorities were on the increase. The number of children being looked after by local authorities in England on 31 March 1997, showed a 2 per cent rise over the previous year and a 5 per cent rise in comparison with 1994 (DoH 1998d). The figures for the year to the end of March 1998 showed a further 4 per cent rise. Within the overall pattern, figures showed a 2,000 increase in the number of care orders taken out by local authorities and an even more dramatic upturn in the number of care orders used for children at the very start of their contact with social services. In 1997/98, 4,600 children started to be looked after under care orders, compared to 3,300 in the previous year (DoH 1998e). Conversely, the number of children starting to be looked after under voluntary agreements fell by 1,500 over the same period.

The difference between the 1997 administration and its predecessors lay in its belief in the more positive part which public action had to play in improving services for children. The case for action continued to be made in a further series of reports which emphasised shortcomings in their care, both within residential and community services. A damning Inspector's Report of services in the London Borough of Ealing, for example, found that the Social Services Department had fallen prey to a 'culture of hopelessness', in which 94 children on the at-risk register and 93 children in care had not been allocated a social worker (DoH 1998f). A Social Services Inspectorate report of children in the care system, *Someone Else's Children* (DoH 1998g), found 'huge variation in standards up and down the country, and in individual cases'. The Minister responsible for children's services responded to the report (DoH 1998h) by suggesting that it gave support to the government's intention to provide 'a root and branch transformation of children's services'. Given the manifest failures of public care it is not, perhaps, surprising that this transformation was to be sought explicitly within the general New Labour mantra of 'what works' – 'what counts is what works', Paul Boateng (DoH 1998i) – rather than by reasserting the benefits of public provision. The basket of services for children was to remain a mixture of public, voluntary and private provision. The difference lay, rather, in the re-affirmed capacity of publicly-funded, guided and regulated effort in bringing about improvement.

The most direct expression of this new approach lay in the *Quality Protects* initiative which was designed, according to the Department of Health, to 'transform the management of children's social services' (DoH 1998j). The policy combined the ingredients which were now familiar in the administration's approach to social service areas. The delivery of services would include a 'partnership at local level, at national level, between local authorities, voluntary bodies and the NHS'. The direct role of government, and the assumption of public responsibility, would be two-fold. Firstly, government would provide extra money – £375 million over three years for children's services. Secondly, it would place additional obligations upon service planners and deliverers – often through the development of National Standards – and then enforce these requirements through more rigorous forms of inspection. By the time the government's White Paper on the future of social services was published in November 1998, the detail of these changes had begun to be formulated. There was to be a new approach to inspection and regulation of children's services, bringing all forms of provision together. In relation to residential care, for example, the White Paper (Chapter 4.36) made it clear that 'the same regulatory system will in principle apply to all children's homes, whether private, voluntary or local authority . . . All homes will be subject to mandatory inspection.' The linking theme of the reforms was one which made explicit the administration's emphasis upon state responsibility. A system was to be devised in which 'the general public can once again have faith in our *public care* system' (Chapter 3.42 – emphasis added).

Community care

The greater willingness which the Labour government of 1997 showed in using public powers was similarly apparent in its approach to the care of older people. In the residential sector the Department of Health announced its decision to increase the level of public scrutiny of private providers of health and nursing care and to transfer the costs of that scrutiny to the private sector. Social services reports on residential homes had been published since 1994. As from January 1998 the government set out its intention that, as the Minister put it (DoH 1998k), 'Homes which look after frail and vulnerable people and clinics which provide private health care should be open and accountable to the public, and inspection findings should be available to anyone who wants them.' Marketisation in the health service had produced 350 establishments registered as independent hospitals and clinics, providing 10,600 beds in England alone in 1995/96. The cost to health authorities and councils of regulating the sector was estimated at some £37.8 million, of which only £16.6 million was recovered in fees. Pointing out that the shortfall was made up by money 'taken away from hospital and community care', the announcement included a 40 per cent increase in registration fees, thus shifting the cost out of the public sector and onto the private providers.

Nor were considerations only financial. The government was also alert to evidence of market failure in social services, particularly in relation to the needs of particular groups. Such difficulties were well illustrated in a 1998 Inspection report of Community Care Services for Black and Minority Ethnic Older People

(DoH 1998l) which concluded that 'there was a distinct lack of choice and many of the services were inappropriate to the needs of black and ethnic minority older people'. Service planners, as well as providers, too often regarded the needs of such users as 'marginal' to their main concerns. The evidence of this report was to prove influential in some of the proposals contained in the November 1998 White Paper, *Modernising Social Services [document 10b]*.

The government's focus within community care, however, was primarily upon the boundary between health and social services and, most particularly within the field of mental health. Here the fall in NHS beds for the mentally ill, and the marketisation of community care, had produced particular concerns in relation to the capacity of the system to respond to patient need and public safety. The introduction of market principles in health and social services had resulted in a rapid increase in private sector mental health nursing homes from 460 in 1991/92 to 1,010 in 1996/97. Such facilities now housed some of the most acutely ill patients in the mental health field. At the end of March 1998, 850 of the 12,000 patients compulsorily detained in mental health facilities in England were held in private mental nursing homes (DoH 1998m). This complex cocktail of split responsibilities and mixed provision produced a policy document, *Modernising Health and Social Services* (DoH 1998n) published in September 1998, in which the Secretary of State declared that 'we will break down the Berlin Wall between health and social care' (DoH 1998o). A series of specific measures included pooled budgets between health and social services, the assignment of a leading role to a single authority in commissioning both social and health care within a locality and integrated provision in which health trusts or social services departments could take responsibility for in-house provision across the range of services. Whereas the break-up of large-scale organisations into independent and competitive components had been a key part of the privatisation approach to public services, the New Labour policy was quite different. Both health and social services departments were once again to become direct providers of a range of ancillary services – such as chiropody or social care – funded and delivered by the public sector. Nevertheless, the language of markets had not entirely disappeared from government discourse. A joint document, signed by Ministers of State responsible for Health and Social Services – *Partnership in Action: New Opportunities for Joint Working between Health and Social Services* (DoH 1998p) – still talked of working together as 'part of the core business' of health and social care. Its emphasis, however, lay upon replacing the competitive relationships of the past with new co-operation: 'Instead of the fragmentation and bureaucracy of the internal market, we are building a system of integrated care, based on partnership. Social services have a key role in that partnership.'

In the community, the gathering pace of community care scandals from that of Christopher Clunis (Ritchie 1994) onwards had already created a climate within the non-institutional care of mentally ill individuals in which use of compulsory powers was on the increase. Formal admission of male patients, for example, rose by 30 per cent between 1991/92 and 1996/97 (DoH 1998q).

The response of the Labour administration was a reassertion of public responsibility in the mental health area, albeit one which again drew significantly on
the social authoritarian strand within the Party's thinking. The earliest initiative
of substance within this field was announced in September 1997 when an
effective halt was called to the further closure of mental hospitals, without the
completion of a stringent new vetting system (DoH 1997c). Speaking at the end
of that year, the Minister responsible, Paul Boateng, drew a distinction between
the new policy approach and that of the previous administration:

> 'We must not forget the impact which the last 18 years has had on mental health services.
> Some progress has been made in developing local services. But the policy focused too
> much on closure and not enough on reprovision. Gaps in mental health services result to
> a large part from chronic under-investment over many years.' (DoH 1997d)

At this stage, the government's response rested mostly on a willingness to accept
a new level of responsibility for the public funding of community mental health
services. The same announcement set out the additional £5 million to be provided to ease the immediate pressure on acute beds and a further £6 million
specifically for mental health services in 1998/99.

The policy changes of 1997, however, were only a prelude to a 'root and
branch' review of mental health legislation instituted in the following year and
predicated upon a 'safety-plus' policy which combined a willingness to devote
greater resources to public provision in this field and a willingness to 'support
compulsory treatment, where deemed necessary for those patients not formally
detained' (DoH 1998r). The policy of community care, which had been pursued for more than thirty years, was formally brought to an end. Secretary of
State Dobson declared directly that 'Care in the community has failed' (DoH
1998s). While there was to be no return to 'locking up mentally ill patients in
long stay institutions', policy was to shift in favour of 'assertive' services, com-
bining additional secure units and 24-hour outreach teams in the community,
equipped with 'compliance orders and community treatment orders to provide
a prompt and effective legal basis to ensure that patients get supervised care if
they do not take their medication or if their condition deteriorates'. In December 1998 the reforms were set out in a strategy document, *Modernising Mental
Health Services* (DoH 1998t). The Foreword by the Secretary of State emphasised
the new compulsory powers which would be available for treating individuals
who posed a threat to themselves and others:

> 'We are going to bring the laws on mental health up-to-date. In particular to ensure that
> patients who might otherwise be a danger to themselves and others are no longer allowed
> to refuse to comply with the treatment they need. We will also be changing the law to
> permit the detention of a small group of people who have not committed a crime but
> whose untreatable psychiatric disorder makes them dangerous.'

The document placed the blame for previous policy failure directly on lack
of investment, suggesting that while community care policies had been identified as a priority, 'the gap between cheap words and a proper commitment to

funding change and reforming services has been glaring'. In contrast, the new policies were to be backed up with a substantial share of the Department of Health's Comprehensive Spending Review money to be devoted to improvements in the field. An additional £700 million over a three-year period would include £500 million directed to changing the way in which services are delivered, £120 million invested in new and effective drug therapies and £70 million in training.

In terms of public and private responsibility, Labour's policy in this area was thus almost a mirror image of that provided by its predecessor. There, libertarian and neo-liberal thinking had forestalled the use of compulsory intervention in the private lives of individuals over whom the state had no control. At the same time, the responsibilities of the state to provide public services for the discharged mental health patient had been minimised, with care left to families or overstretched community services. Labour's policy set out to extend public responsibility in both directions. Public services would be improved, while powers to intervene compulsorily in the lives of private citizens would be extended.

Modernising social services

The early policy-making of the incoming New Labour ministry in relation to social services culminated in the publication of its November 1998 White Paper *Modernising Social Services [document 10b]*. The paper combined a series of strands in the government's approach to the division of responsibilities between the public and private spheres. On the one hand, it demonstrated a willingness to intervene in the social services market which had developed under the requirements of the Community Care Act. On the other, it endorsed the ideological indifference which the government generally claimed in relation to issues of structure and ownership. For example, Chapter 7 of the White Paper, 'Public and Private Sector Provision', declares that, 'Best value must be secured in all social services, whether provided in-house or contracted out to the voluntary or private sector. This Government does not take an ideological approach to this issue, and has no preconceptions about whether the public or the voluntary or private sector should be the preferred providers.'

At the same time, however, indifference to ideology extended to a rejection of 'the last Government's devotion to privatisation of care provision [which] put dogma before users' interests, and threatened a fragmentation of vital services'. The White Paper identified a series of specific criticisms of the marketisation project in the personal social services. These included underlying problems of *eligibility* – 'Decisions about who gets services and who does not are often unclear, and vary from place to place' – and *equity* – 'Many people feel that the care system is not fair. There are variations in who gets what services, inconsistencies in what types of provision are available in different parts of the country, and differences in how charging works.' From these causes, practical problems also followed. The White Paper highlighted the concentration of community care services on fewer users:

'This means that some people who would benefit from purposeful intervention at a lower level of service . . . are not receiving any support. This increases the risk that they in turn become more likely to need much more complicated levels of support as their independence is compromised. That is good neither for the individual nor, ultimately, for the social services, the NHS and the taxpayer'

and problems over charging for services. Discretionary charges for home care, meals on wheels, day centre places and so on were a particular cause for concern, illustrated by what the White Paper called a 'random example' in which, in different local authority areas, 'someone with a weekly income of £115 and receiving 12 hours of care per week could pay £13 a week in one area and £48 per week in the other'.

In response to these criticisms, *Modernising Social Services* set out a series of policy proposals. The principle underlying the New Labour approach was identified in the first section of the document:

'Social services are for all of us. We all depend on good social services to be there at such times of crisis, to help in making the right decisions and working out what needs to be done. Social services, therefore, do not just support a small number of "social casualties", they are an important part of the fabric of a caring society. It is a concern for everyone that social services should be providing the best possible service.'

This bold statement of universality marked a deliberate contrast with the social services reform proposals published in the last weeks of the previous government *[document 10a]*, where the emphasis had been placed upon private and family responsibility, with public provision relegated to a residual and supportive role. Labour's claimed indifference to ideology meant that the new policy relied for reframing the debate about public and private upon 'partnership' and regulation as the way forward. Secretary of State, Frank Dobson, introducing the White Paper (DoH 1998u) emphasised that the proposals would 'ensure that local councils, the NHS, voluntary bodies and commercial providers work together to help people live independent and fulfilling lives'. Over the whole sector, however, new regulators with substantial powers would 'cover all services, no matter who provides them'. These arrangements were to include Regional Commissioners for Care Standards for regulating care services, with 'tough new powers and national standards'; a General Social Care Council, responsible for raising professional and training standards and new arrangements for performance management in social services, 'based on the Best Value regime, with national performance standards and targets'.

Specifically, the White Paper promised an expansion of the direct payments scheme of its predecessors, a new national scheme for charging for services, reducing variation and introducing 'greater transparency and fairness in the contribution that people are asked to make towards their social care', and a levelling of the playing field between public, voluntary and private provision.

10.2 Health policies

Of all the social policy areas discussed in this book, the National Health Service remains the one with which the Labour Party has been most identified, and to which it has been most attached both in office and in opposition. In government after 1997 it has proved to be the policy field in which the privatising and marketising legacy of the Conservative years has been most directly addressed and, to some extent, reversed. Eighteen months into office, for example, analysts were reporting that ten private hospitals had closed since 1996 and that a further 50 were expected to follow suit over the next few years as a result of improvements in NHS care, rising premiums and a reversal of tax breaks for insurance payments introduced during the Conservative years (*Independent on Sunday* 6 September 1998). Yet, as Bartlett *et al.* (1998: 2) suggest, 'despite the rhetoric concerning "the abolition of the internal market", key features of the quasi-market are to be retained, including the purchaser–provider split and GP-led commissioning'.

While policy results were mixed, rhetorically – and unlike other areas, such as education, where the new administration went out of its way to emphasise support for private provision – Health Ministers talked openly of restoring to the public sphere a series of activities which had been shifted in the opposite direction. Among the tasks handed to an early savings Task Force (DoH 1997e), for example, was consideration of whether some of the '£500 million health authorities and Trusts spend each year with the private sector . . . could be better spent with the NHS'. A practical demonstration of the superiority of public over private provision followed, in the summer of 1998, when it was announced (DoH 1998v) that commercial insurance against non-clinical risk by individual Trusts was to be replaced by a pooled arrangement within the NHS as a whole. A survey by the NHS Executive had revealed that Trusts were spending some £55 million a year on premiums in all categories of commercial insurance, in return for paid claims of only some £10–11 million. The case for public arrangements was expressed by the Minister, Alan Milburn, in this way:

> 'Much of the money ends up as profit for the insurance companies at the expense of frontline patient services. Competition in the NHS has been deeply inefficient. By co-operating, NHS Trusts will help save the National Health Service up to £45 million a year for investment in frontline patient care. In the new NHS cooperation and efficiency go hand in glove. Today's announcement is one more nail in the coffin of the expensive and discredited NHS internal market.'

When, during the autumn of 1998, research evidence indicated that, across a range of measures, satisfaction with the health service in Britain out-ran that in the United States, Australia, Canada and New Zealand, while costing less per head of the population than in any of these, Frank Dobson was able to tell an international symposium in Washington that the tax-based NHS was more efficient and more popular than any primarily private-based alternative (DoH 1998w).

Even when obliged, by the government's overall spending limits, to raise charges, the health administration attempted to do so in a way which placed a clear distance between itself and the enthusiasm for charging which had marked its predecessor. When the annual round of prescription charges had to be met in March 1998, Labour ministers attempted to weather the inevitable storm by announcing the first real-terms fall in charges since 1981 (DoH 1998x). In April 1998, the Secretary of State went on record to rule out charges for the 'hotel' elements of hospital stays, consulting family doctors or for contraceptive pills. All these suggestions had been raised during the Comprehensive Spending Review, but were now rejected because, Mr Dobson said, 'charging would break the principle that people should have access to health care when they need it' (*The Independent* 1 April 1998). Nonetheless, some decisions by the new government – to start charging for travel vaccines and to transfer the costs of treatment in the case of road accidents to insurance companies – suggested that the division between public and private responsibility had not been unambiguously resolved in favour of the former. In the case of travel vaccines, the government were able to argue that these were costs voluntarily entered into by relatively well-off individuals. The amounts of money, however, were not trivial. The Department of Health estimated that a single traveller would face charges of between £100 and £150, while the cost to a family might amount to £500 (*Sunday Telegraph* 12 July 1998). In the case of road accident costs, the Road Traffic (NHS Charges) Bill of November 1998 emphasised the government's intention to use the Compensation Recovery Unit of the Benefits Agency to recoup money from insurance companies where road accidents resulted in out-patient or in-patient treatment. The initiative was vulnerable to charges that the decision contributed to a shift towards insurance-based health care, in which the individual would pay through increased premiums.

Openness

The commercialisation of professional relationships, and the introduction of private sector methods and money into the health service brought with them, during the early 1990s, an increased emphasis upon confidentiality in relation to health service transactions and, in terms of the basic focus of this book, a growing tendency for public bodies to conduct their business in private session. The New Labour health administration moved to redress this transfer from public scrutiny to private safety in a number of areas. In June 1997 details of all PFI projects with a capital value of more than £1 million were placed wholly in the public domain (DoH 1997f). In the same month, the Secretary of State announced his intention to place regulations before Parliament in order to guarantee that Board Meetings of NHS Trusts should be open to the public (DoH 1997g). When the parliamentary procedure was finally completed on 6 February 1998, Trust Board meetings became obliged to be open to the public; advertised in advance, open to media reporting and required to treat any sub-committee proceedings in the same way. In the meantime, gagging clauses which had been placed in the contracts of NHS staff, preventing individuals from speaking publicly on matters of concern, had been removed. The capacity of NHS bodies to deny one another information on the grounds of commercial confidentiality was also abolished. The Minister responsible, Alan Milburn, provided the link which allied these changes with broader policy thrusts within the Ministry (DoH 1997h):

> 'The culture of secrecy is often an excuse to avoid accountability and has no place in the modern NHS.
>
> 'The divisive internal market has resulted in NHS bodies classifying and secreting away information for no reason. In the past, NHS Trusts frequently withheld in-year financial information, hindering Health Authorities in the sensible planning of local health services. The government is dismantling the internal market. In place of competition the NHS will work together for the benefit of patients.'

GP fundholding

Of greater practical importance in the abolition of the internal market was reform of the GP Fundholding scheme. Less than three weeks after being elected, the new administration deferred the eighth wave of funding applications to join the existing scheme in 1998/99 (DoH 1997i). Figures from the Department of Health suggested that in 60 per cent of Health Authorities in England, patients of fundholding GPs were, on average, admitted to hospital more quickly than non-fundholding GPs (DoH 1997j). A series of reforms to those arrangements were introduced in order to ensure that patients of non-fundholders were not disadvantaged by the financial arrangements applying in the fundholding scheme. These included a new power for Health Authorities to adjust fundholder budgets where calls upon their own funds for emergency activity would otherwise have had to be found by cutting back on services for non-fundholder patients. The new Secretary of State also issued a series of instructions that, as from April 1998, hospitals would no longer be able to set different waiting time standards between GP fundholder and Health Authority patients, and that admission for urgent and non-urgent treatments should be on the basis of clinical priority, regardless of the status of the patient's GP. In other words, Trusts were not to offer preferential admission to the patients of GP fundholders and fundholders were not to press for faster treatment except on clinical or social grounds. In relation to the central concerns of this text, the reforms strengthened the hand of the Health Authority as provider of services, as against the advantages which had previously been available to individual GP purchasers.

The same announcement of amendments to existing Fundholder arrangements also contained the first formal indication of the new administration's approach to future primary health care plans. New commissioning arrangements were to be put in place which would emphasise co-operation, rather than competition for the purpose of ensuring that patients had equal access to health care based on their clinical needs (DoH 1997k). Pilot schemes were set up, to begin on 1 April 1998 and based upon GP Commissioning Groups (GPCGs). The new groups were to encompass a range of primary care professionals, working together with the local health authority to commission health care for their patients and taking responsibility for their own prescribing budget. Some twenty pilot schemes were envisaged in the original announcement, but in September 1997, 42 were actually announced (DoH 1997l), following what Frank Dobson called 'overwhelming enthusiasm for this new model of delivering local health services'.

The confirmation of pilot schemes was accompanied by further amendments to existing fundholder arrangements which, essentially, re-emphasised the need for individual fundholders to act consistently within the overall plans of Health Authorities and which further reined back the financial freedoms of fundholders, where these could be shown to act to the detriment of non-fundholder patients. The Government was at pains to emphasise its intention to steer a middle path between the command-and-control model of the 1970s and what it called the 'market free for all of the early 1990s'. Commissioning pilots would be provided with flexibility and choice but would operate within a framework of partnership and cooperation, rather than market relations.

The same emphasis was clearly to the fore in another of the initiatives which formed part of a wider approach by the New Labour administration. The possibility of Action Zones in health care was announced by Frank Dobson in June 1997, when he emphasised their potential contribution to the new NHS ethos of co-operative partnership, combined with another over-arching theme, that of tackling health inequalities through a new public health strategy (DoH 1997m). In his words:

'We have got to get every part of the NHS working together. We simply can't afford some of the wasteful crack-pot competition that the internal market provoked at the outset. I know as a result of the bitter experience of competition, the idea of co-operation is making a comeback.'

Health Action Zones would need to show a capacity to bring together a range of health interests, together with those in housing, education, employment and industry which produce an impact upon health and ill-health. By February 1998 bids had been received from 49 of the 100 English Health Authority areas (DoH 1998y), leading to the establishment of eleven zones during 1998/99. £5.3 million in 1998/99 and £30 million in the following year was to be made available in order to advance what the Secretary of State described as 'the cornerstone of our public health strategy – our commitment to drive up the standards of health amongst the poorest in our country at a faster rate than for the general population'. When a further announcement led to the doubling of the number of zones (DoH 1998z), covering both rural and inner city areas at a cost of an additional £15 million, Mr Dobson again emphasised the importance of the initiative in overcoming barriers between health and local authorities, and between professionals in areas of high deprivation. The emphasis upon addressing inequality, and prioritising the needs of the least well off, marks out the policy as quite different from the focus of the previous fifteen years, most especially in its belief in the capacity of public effort to bring about such objectives. It stands in contrast, too, to a number of the zonal policies developed in other social policy areas of the same government, where – as in education, for example – the emphasis appeared to be far more upon cutting across local public authorities and enhancing market conditions of choice and diversity than upon strong public effort on behalf of the most disadvantaged.

Internal markets, competition and equity

Among the very first actions of the incoming Labour administration in health was the announcement of the abolition of the internal market which had been the central creation of the neo-liberal marketeers during the last period of Conservative administration. Announcing the change, the new Secretary of State, Frank Dobson, concentrated upon two aspects of the market, its inefficiency and inequity (DoH 1997n). In his words:

'There are examples galore where the so-called "internal market", in which GP fundholders and health authorities buy services from NHS Trusts, has led to a two-tier health service. The NHS cannot truly be called national unless every man, woman and child in the country has equal access to high-quality treatment, and unless the speed with which they receive that treatment is governed solely by their clinical condition rather than the size of their GP's budget.

'But we remain committed to ending the internal market in health care, which has placed so many patients at a disadvantage. We must also undo the damage the market has created – the never-ending paperchase of invoices, and the flawed measures of efficiency which concentrate on numbers of patients being treated rather than the outcome of their treatment.'

Within the new policy, a wholly fresh impetus was applied to the notion that openness and co-operation should replace what was seen as the rivalry, secretiveness, divisiveness and fragmentation of the competitive market. The object of co-operation was to be equality of outcome, in which the health of the poorest individuals was to be raised to that of their better-off contemporaries. The vocabulary of fairness and equity re-entered the health arena, permeating a whole range of initiatives and particularly those which sought to bring a public health agenda to the forefront of policy making.

The 1997 Labour Government appointed Tessa Jowell as a Minister with specific responsibility for public health. She described her title (DoH 1997o) as marking

'a new approach to health – setting our mission to tackle the inequalities that give rise to ill-health alongside the service that treats us when we are ill. . . . The evidence is compelling that people who live in disadvantaged circumstances have more illness, greater distress, and shorter lives than those who are more affluent. . . . We will wage war on inequalities where children's health is determined by the accident of their birth. . . . For

177

this Government the health of the individual cannot be separated from the surrounding environment, and improvements in individual health mean action which involves the wider community.'

The contrast with the policy of the previous administration, and its strategy document *The Health of the Nation*, was thus clearly marked out. In focusing upon diseases and services, the previous policy had placed the responsibility for good health squarely upon individuals and lifestyles. Structural health inequalities played no part in the thinking of the free marketeers. In the terms with which we are concerned in this book, Labour's health approach involved a reaffirmation of the health consequences of public rather than private agencies and activities, emphasising the communal benefits to be derived from co-operative effort across the range of public policy areas. Research evidence which drew attention to inequalities once again found its way into the public domain, with policy conclusions clearly underlined. When the Office for National Statistics published its Decennial Supplement on Health Inequalities in September 1997 (DoH 1997p), for example, Minister Jowell commented:

'This report tells the tale of two Britains divided by ever widening health inequality. It shows the stark reality of a nation divided by its health, i.e. the poorer and more socially deprived you are, the more likely you are to suffer ill-health and die younger than those higher up the social scale.'

In terms of practical action, the new focus upon tackling inequalities in health led to a series of announcements. In September 1997 (DoH 1997q), the Government undertook an exercise to redistribute NHS funds to better reflect the health needs of local communities, explicitly stating that the intention was 'to better focus NHS resources on tackling health inequalities, and consider concerns that the existing funding formula fails to do so'.

When Baroness Jay addressed a regional conference of health service interests in September 1997 (DoH 1997r) she drew together the themes of quality and inequality and the interlocking efforts of the curative and public health policies of the administration. The speech revolved around a repudiation of the whole notion of privatisation in the health service: 'The NHS may be a multibillion pound enterprise but it is not making widgets or selling financial services – it's not a business answerable to shareholders for a profit margin.' Instead, the principles of equity and access were to be 'central to the NHS quality agenda – as it is to the government's drive to tackle health inequalities. This is when our NHS policies and our public health policies come together. The two are inseparable.'

One of the most practical areas in which the new principles were quickly applied was to be found in dentistry which, under the charging and other reforms of the Conservative health policies had ceased, in large parts of the country, to provide a public service of any reliability. In successive announcements during the year after May 1997, additional money and new initiatives were applied to the development of new public provision, especially in relation to children and areas of health inequality. In March 1998, for example, a further £10 million was announced (DoH 1998aa), in addition to £19 million of new money which had been committed during the previous nine months. The March money followed fresh research evidence which emphasised the pattern of consistently higher levels of tooth decay in the economically poorer Health Authority areas. The number of decayed, missing or filled teeth of five-year-olds in the deprived areas was found to be some 40 per cent higher than elsewhere, while children aged between three and five years in deprived areas were 10 per cent less likely to attend the dentist than their counterparts. Using recognised deprivation indices, the £10 million was targeted through local authority council wards, providing additional payments for work with children under six to dentists whose practice addresses fell within these areas. As a result, both access to services and equality of outcome were to be enhanced.

Spending

There is no space in this section for a detailed account of public spending initiatives in the health field after May 1997. The PFI initiatives discussed in relation to housing and education were repeated here, also, albeit without the uncritical celebration of private sector involvement which was more character-istic elsewhere. In health, Ministers were more at pains to stress the unsatis-factory nature of their inheritance. While education circulars called on local authorities to make their bids more attractive to the private sector, health policy emphasised the need for public priorities to take precedence over private inter-ests. The Minister responsible, Alan Milburn, set out the new thinking in this way (DoH 1997s):

'The PFI situation in Health inherited by this Government is a total mess. PFI has manifestly failed to deliver the goods. . . . Time and money have been spent wrestling with apparently insurmountable problems and an immature market place has been left to run out of control. . . .

'Future capital schemes in the NHS will be driven by patients' needs rather than how attractive they are to the private sector . . . new arrangements will put health need, not market whim, in the driving seat when deciding where hospitals should be built. Previ-ously the whims of the market determined capital development plans in the NHS. In the future new hospitals will be built where they are needed most, and where they will deliver the greatest benefit to patients.'

Within the new PFI arrangements, Labour introduced a distinction between services, such as catering, cleaning, laundry and pathology, and the construc-tion and maintenance of actual buildings. The PFI arrangements were to apply to the latter, leaving the service element to be provided through the public sector. Nevertheless, criticisms of the PFI project were felt in the health service, as in other parts of government. Short-term gains to the capital spending pro-gramme were being achieved at the expense of higher costs in the longer term.

Senior consultants called for a halt to the programme, because the revenue implications of paying for the new building costs were putting local health services at risk. The *Financial Times*, in June 1998, reported an analysis by management consultants Kingsley Manning which suggested that each PFI deal would cost an additional £200 million over and above the costs of direct public capital spending, creating the loss of up to 1,000 jobs among clinical staff and in reduced capacity in hospitals and community services.

Outside the PFI, the health service gained more than any other social policy area from the new Government's positive belief in the benefits to be derived from public expenditure. Although outside the main scope of this book, much of the pressure upon Labour's health policy derived from a specific 'early' Manifesto pledge to reduce hospital waiting lists by 100,000. The Government came to office against the background of growing lists which, accountancy firm Chantrey Vellacott estimated were set to increase by 340,000 over the next year because of three previous years of low real terms increases in NHS funding. The report concluded that an extra £20 billion would be necessary over the next three years to keep waiting lists at their current level and prevent further rises (reported in the *Daily Mail* 3 March 1997). Ironically, the BMA suggested that pressure to reduce waiting lists was increasing the number of contracts placed with private hospitals, in order to cut the longest lists (*The Times* 25 July 1998).

It was within this context that, despite the self-imposed limitations on spending over the first two years of the administration, the first Budget released £1.2 billion from reserves for health spending across the UK. In a determined attempt to avoid the winter crises which had become a regular feature of the health service over previous years, a further £300 million followed in October (DoH 1997t), together with a reallocation of £100 million which, the Government said, had been saved through efficiency savings and its reforms to the internal market. An allocation of an additional £300 million followed before the end of the year, through the reform of the National Lottery (DoH 1997u). A national network of healthy living centres was to be set up, concentrated upon areas where basic facilities were in short supply. Finally, in 1997 a further £80 million was allocated for the following financial year (DoH 1997v), to be brought about through cuts in NHS management costs. The Government had come into office promising to move £1 billion from bureaucracy into patient care during the course of the Parliament. This commitment had been repeated in the December 1997 White Paper *The New NHS – Modern, Dependable*. The document emphasised the Government's intention to move away from the marketising policies of the early 1990s. It proposed the end of the internal market and the phased replacement of different purchasing arrangements to a uniform system of 500 Primary Care Groups (PCGs), each covering a 'natural community' of some 100,000 people. Mays and Dixon (1998: 198), whose calculations suggest that the new PCGs will replace up to 5,000 existing purchasing arrangements – health authorities, fundholders, locality-based commissioning groups and so on – identify the main purpose of the change as the Government's wish to create greater equity in health service delivery. In order to do so, the White Paper affirmed the benefits of direct spending on public services and set the face of the new administration against the managerialism which had formed a central tenet of New Right practice. While reservations remained about the consistency of some proposals – reconciling decentralising initiatives with the 'one nation' approach, for example – it seemed clear, as Bartlett *et al.* (1998: 13) conclude, that the White Paper represented 'a significant movement away from the individualisation of welfare to an acceptance of the deeper structural issues that determine healthcare'.

In the same month as the £80 million savings were announced, the Minister responsible told a conference of health service managers that, 'Decisions about how best to use resources for patient care are best made by those who treat patients' (DoH 1997w). Under Labour, doctors and nurses were to be in the NHS driving seat. Even here, however, Labour took action to emphasise the public responsibilities of health service workers. The *Sunday Times* reported on 10 May 1998 that the contracts of Britain's 23,000 hospital consultants were to be rewritten in order to limit the amount of private work undertaken by them. 'Ministers are alarmed', said the newspaper, 'by the findings of a new report which revealed that the proportion of earnings from private work doubled from 25 to 50 per cent between 1983 and 1994'.

In support of its general policy of bearing down upon managerialism, the bulk of the December 1997 savings were to be found directly from management costs – £12 million from the Health Authorities, £36 million from Trust management costs and £25 million from GP Fundholder management allowances. The scepticism towards the managerialism of the former regime was increased, in April 1998, with the publication of a Department of Health report which suggested that the management costs of NHS Trusts had been artificially underestimated in the first half of the 1990s by the non-inclusion of contract services management costs. The Department suggested that £100 million had been removed from the acknowledged costs to the Trusts in this way, creating 'perverse incentives' for trust managers to use private companies for services such as cleaning and laundry (*The Guardian* 4 April 1998).

During 1998 the March Budget provided a further additional £500 million, specifically targeted at reducing hospital waiting lists which, despite the Manifesto promise, had risen stubbornly during Labour's first year in office. The concentration upon waiting lists was accompanied by claims that it began to cause distortions in patterns of treatment as hospitals concentrated upon patients who could be quickly removed from the lists, rather than those in greatest need (*The Independent* 19 March 1998). The fiftieth anniversary of the NHS and the results of the Comprehensive Spending Review both took place during July 1998. A new ring-fenced Modernisation Fund was set up, with £5 billion set aside for targeted improvement in services. £1.2 billion of this was committed during the first year, 1999/2000, including £49 million for Health Action Zones. Overall, the CSR produced an additional £20 billion to be spent on the health services over three years, contributing to an average 4 per cent increase in real terms in all English Health Authority budgets during the first twelve months (DoH 1998bb).

Labour's commitment to a public health care system, free at the point of use and directed by the pursuit of equity in health outcomes, emerged as the strongest theme in this social policy area, despite continuing difficulties over waiting lists, rationing of particular treatments by individual Trusts and ever-present demands for more resources. The extent to which the new administration had departed from the policies of its predecessor might be gauged from calls which were still made from the Conservative opposition. *The Times* of 11 June 1998 carried a report of a call from former MP Michael Portillo for a larger role for private health care in Britain as the 'only way' to increase national spending in this area. He accused all political parties of regarding the NHS as 'sacred and untouchable' and therefore outside the scope of necessary reform. To a more modest extent the same sentiments were echoed by the shadow Health Minister, Ann Widdicombe, when addressing the 1998 Conservative Party Conference. She called for the guilt to be removed from people who wanted to choose their own provider of health care. In a novel reformulation of what had, traditionally, been described as queue-jumping she declared, 'there is nothing morally repugnant about supplying your own health: you are freeing up the NHS to look after somebody else' (*The Guardian* 7 October 1998). The idea that private was best, and public came second was thus still alive and being promoted in mainstream political thinking.

The account provided in this book has tended to overemphasise the compartmentalisation of social policy between different government departments. In fact, as the public health policies discussed here particularly illustrate, activity in one sphere of administration can have important consequences for others. The pensions mis-selling scandals of 1988–94, for example, occupied the attention of health service Ministers in the new government as part of a general attack upon the recalcitrance of pension companies in addressing the difficulties caused. In May 1997 the Personal Investment Authority reported that some 570,000 people had been identified as having been left worse off as a result of the scandal. Of all occupational sectors, the NHS had the largest single proportion of people who had been mis-sold private pensions, with evidence emerging of sales staff appearing within hospital wards in pursuit of the policies of the then-government. The Department estimated (DoH 1997x) that, on information provided by pensions companies, up to 30,000 people could be involved. By August 1997 only 200 cases had been resolved and further groups of individuals had been identified as disadvantaged. When the pace of redress failed to quicken, the Department of Health introduced a new deposit scheme of its own, in order to allow NHS staff immediate reinstatement into the service's own pension plan (DoH 1997y) Up to 42,000 staff were now anticipated to qualify as priority cases for reinstatement.

The private pensions scandal, and the actions of the Health Ministers in providing a public sector solution, illustrate the very different set of beliefs under which this Ministry was directed by the Labour Government of May

1997. In general terms, privatisation and marketisation were rejected as part of the solution contemporary health care needs. In their place, the essential public service tenets of equality, cooperation and redistribution were once again powerfully in evidence.

10.3 Conclusions

There are no grand conclusions with which this book can end. As suggested at the outset, the debate between public and private responsibility in social policy and social welfare is one in which protagonists have been continuously engaged. The emerging ideas of New Labour are thus a contribution to a process which is never settled and always evolving. Indeed, for many commentators (see, for example, Jacques 1998) the continuities between New Labour and the old Conservative regimes are more striking than the differences. Hall (1998: 11) summarises this viewpoint in relation to the policies which have been the focus of this text when he describes New Labour's approach as dominated by 'the deregulation of markets, the wholesale refashioning of the public sector by the New Managerialism, the continued privatisation of public assets, low taxation, breaking the "inhibitions" to market flexibility, institutionalising the culture of private provision and personal risk, and privileging in its moral discourse the values of self sufficiency, competitiveness and entrepreneurial dynamism.'

Nevertheless, in comparison with the period between 1979 and 1997, when privatisation and marketisation were so heavily promoted as holding the key to policy and practice, the account set out here of the period post May 1997 suggests some important contrasts and distinctions.

Most decisively, as Bartlett *et al.* (1998: 1) conclude, the approach taken by the new government is 'not as focused on market solutions or as ideologically driven as that of the previous administration'. Indeed, a positive pride in ideological indifference is one of the strongest themes which binds the different social welfare ministries of New Labour together. Of course, such a claim is not to be taken at face value. Such an emphatic disavowal of ideology is itself indicative of an approach which goes beyond simple pragmatism. In Labour's own terms, the positive willingness to combine elements from previous approaches – the state and the market – represents a Third Way.

Within that Third Way, some common characteristics can be identified. For a government determined to scotch the 'tax and spend' legacy of its own Party, Labour in office has delivered a greater degree of redistribution by stealth than the public presentation of its programmes might suggest. In each of the areas considered in these final chapters, a common belief emerges in the power of public spending to address the problems faced by Ministers. As Hills (1998: 25) suggests, even after the public relations hype has been sifted,

'the reallocation of resources involved implies spending on health and education running at a combined level more than £5 billion a year higher by the end of the period than they would have done if the distribution of government spending had remained unchanged. This is roughly equivalent to what would have been raised by putting up income tax rates by 2p in the pound.'

Belief in the positive potential of public expenditure is not uniformly matched, however, by a similarly strong belief that services purchased by state spending should be state-provided. While the emphasis varies between the different policy areas considered here, all include examples of service delivery in which private, rather than public, providers have been preferred. For the most part, however, private sector involvement is incorporated within an environment in which the state system strives to provide a high-quality service, on a universal basis. This outcome is most unequivocally to be found within the policies promoted by the Ministry of Health, both in relation to social services and the National Health Services. In education, while neo-liberal thinking has been considerably more influential, the result has still been, as Hills (1998: 33) puts it, 'to rule out a retreat to a privatised safety net'. 'Partnership' is New Labour's key word to describe the public and private mix in service delivery. The advantages claimed for competitive markets have, for the most part, been set aside in favour of the benefits which collaboration is expected to deliver.

Only in the field of social security has there been a major shift away from the essentially universalist approach, in favour of an expanded private welfare system and a retreat in state responsibility towards a means-tested residualism. The private pension plans favoured in the Green Paper of December 1998 clearly envisage a future in which self-provision will play a far greater role and in which the market, rather than the collective arrangements of Beveridge, will have to take the strain of providing for future generations. Even here, however, as Roberts et al. (1998: 275) summarise it, 'the evidence so far suggests that the emphasis on individual responsibility for welfare will continue but with greater emphasis on equity and participation and a recognition of the structural aspects of social well-being'.

This recognition of structural forces, beyond the individual, marks a fundamental difference between the approach of the post-May 1997 period and that of the previous administration. It found one of its most comprehensive expressions in the response of the Health Secretary to the Acheson *Report into Inequalities in Health* (Acheson 1998) *[document 15]*, in which Frank Dobson set out a synthesis of the different initiatives across government departments which might produce an impact upon structurally produced health inequalities. More broadly, in response to structural issues, the New Labour attitude to service delivery – in both public and private forms – places a far greater emphasis upon state regulation and oversight than envisaged by its free market predecessors. Whiteside (1998: 216) provides a warning from the experience of inter-war health markets that while 'on the surface, public regulation of private provision appears to be a cheap and effective way of securing comprehensive cover, in practice it has proved anything but'. Nevertheless, the 'tough' side of Labour's policy tenderness has been consistently applied in the language which Ministers use in describing central government oversight of service delivery. In some areas, such as education and social services, the emphasis has been upon greater levels of direct inspection of the performance of street-level providers – teachers and social workers – and greater willingness to intervene when standards of performance are found wanting. In others, the emphasis has been upon a more systemic regulation, with the pension reforms, for example, highlighting 'better regulation to restore confidence in the system'.

Of course, in relation to the theme of this text, the substitution of regulation for direct provision represents a diminution in the public domain. Fitzpatrick (1998: 25), for example, suggests that the substitution of a regulatory state for the welfare state which offered a collective guarantee of security, represents a 'deliberate lowering of individuals' expectations so that they correspond to the requirements of a supervisory, fee-paying state'. Yet, across the range of social welfare services, a linking theme emerges strongly in the actions of the new administration. If privatisation was about rolling back the frontiers of the state, New Labour's approach rested upon a consistent willingness to roll forward the state's requirements in relation to services, through regulation and inspection.

Finally, some consideration should be given to the impact of these policies at the level of individual service users. As already noted, the approach of the administration represented, as Bartlett *et al.* (1998: 13) put it, 'a significant movement away from the individualisation of welfare to an acceptance of the deeper structural issues'. At the micro-level, the same authors nevertheless suggest that 'debates begun by the Conservative administration, on user charges [and] restricting the range of services to be provided free of charge . . . will continue'. The evidence provided in these chapters suggests that, where such decisions have been taken, the basis has been rather different. For the privatisers and marketeers, user charges were positive measures, designed to set clear market signals and assist market actors in making informed choices. For the administration of May 1997, increasing charges – both in terms of scope and amount – was a necessary evil, to be entered into reluctantly and generally avoided.

At another level, however, the evidence presented here suggests that the individualisation of welfare was not consistently reversed by New Labour. The social authoritarianism apparent in a series of areas translates itself into policies which mark a significant shift away from the non-judgemental and universal minimum standards approach upon which the 1945 settlement was more clearly based. Earlier chapters suggested that the reforms of the Conservative years resulted in a privatisation of the consequences of social policy changes in which individual losers within market systems were left to bear those consequences in their private lives. Under New Labour too, but for rather different reasons, a set of individuals emerge as deliberately beyond the boundary of state-accepted responsibility. The bargain proposed by the Prime Minister in his post-election Aylesbury estate speech *[document 11]* was clearly put:

'The basis of this modern civic society is an ethic of mutual responsibility or duty. It is something for something. A society where we play by the rules. You only take out if you put in. That's the bargain.'

Yet, the partnerships and co-operative relationships upon which Labour relies, for example in housing and education, emerge, on closer consideration, as almost exclusively partnerships of the powerful – the police, the local authorities and other outposts of government. In combination, they are better able to promote the behavioural conformities which the Act requires, and to enforce the consequences upon those who fail to oblige. The result of what Hall (1998: 13) describes as this 'low-flying authoritarianism' is to create a group for whom the criminal law, rather than social policy, becomes the main arm of state response.

The choice between the organisation of social welfare services through markets and privatisation on the one hand, or collective social provision on the other, thus embodies a series of fundamental differences. An amalgam of economic, social, political and philosophical stances produce the social policies which emerge on either side of this great divide. While fixing the relative scopes of state and individual responsibility will always, as this text has argued, remain the subject of amendment and debate, the outcomes are profoundly important. Social solidarity and the life-chance of individuals are enhanced or damaged by the decisions made in the policy areas recounted here. As a new century looms, the discussion and determination of these issues remains as alive and as important as it ever has been.

PART FOUR

Chapter 11

DOCUMENTS

Extract from *Social Insurance and Allied Services*, the Beveridge Report (1942), London, HMSO, in which Beveridge sets out the case for compulsory, collective insurance.

(para. 2) 'The schemes of social insurance and allied services which the Interdepartmental Committee have been called on to survey have grown piecemeal. . . .'

(para. 3) 'In all this change and development, each problem has been dealt with separately, with little or no reference to allied problems . . . social insurance and allied services, as they exist today, are conducted by a complex of disconnected administrative organs, proceeding on different principles, doing invaluable service but at a cost in money and trouble and anomalous treatment of identical problems for which there is no justification.'

(para. 5) 'It is not open to question that, by closer co-ordination, the existing social services could be made at once more beneficial and more intelligible to those whom they service and more economical in their administration.'

(para. 9) '. . . social security must be achieved by co-operation between the State and the individual. The State should offer security for service and contribution. The State in organising security should not stifle incentive, opportunity and responsibility; in establishing a national minimum, it should leave room and encouragement for voluntary action by each individual to provide more than that minimum for himself and his family.'

(para. 12) 'Abolition of want requires, first, improvement of State insurance, that is to say provision against interruption and loss of earning power. . . . To prevent interruption or destruction of earning power from leading to want, it is necessary to improve the present schemes of social insurance in three directions: by extension of scope to cover persons now excluded, by extension of purposes to cover risks now excluded, and by raising the rates of benefit.'

(para. 26) '. . . it has been found to accord best with the sentiments of the British people that in insurance organised by the community by use of compulsory powers each individual should stand in on the same terms; none should claim to pay less because he is healthier or has more regular employment. In accord with that view, the proposals of the Report marks another step forward to the development of State insurance as a new type of human institution, differing both from the former methods of preventing or alleviating distress and from voluntary insurance. The terms "social insurance" to describe this institution implies both that it is compulsory and that men stand together with their fellows.'

Document 2

Extract from Aneurin Bevan's *In Place of Fear* (1952) in which he sets out the case for the National Health Service.

'The field in which the claims of individual commercialism come into most immediate conflict with reputable notions of social values in that of health. . . . In this sphere values which are in essence Socialist challenge and win victory after victory against the assertions and practice of the competitive society.

'Modern communities have been made tolerable by the behaviour patterns imposed upon them by the activities of the sanitary inspector and the medical officer of health . . . the whole significance of their contribution is its insistence that the claims of the individual shall subordinate themselves to social codes that have the collective well-being for their aim, irrespective of the extent to which this frustrates individual greed. . . . It would be a fanatical supporter of the competitive society who asserted that the work done in the field of preventative medicine shows the enslavement of the individual to what has come to be described in the United States as "statism". . . .

'Society becomes more wholesome, more serene, and spiritually healthier, if it knows that its citizens have at the back of their consciousness, the knowledge that not only themselves, but all their fellows, have access, when ill, to the best that medical skill can provide. But private charity and endowment, although inescapably essential at one time, cannot meet the cost of all this. If the job is to be done, the state must accept financial responsibility . . .

'Whatever may be said for private insurance, it would be out of place in a national scheme. . . . Limited benefits for limited contributions ignore the overriding consideration that the full range of health machinery must be there in any case, independent of the patient's right of free access to it . . .

'The essence of a satisfactory health service is that the rich and the poor are treated alike, that poverty is not a disability, and wealth is not advantaged. . . .

'A free health service is pure Socialism and as such it is opposed to the hedonism of capitalist society. To call it something for nothing is absurd because everything has to be paid for in some way or another. . . .

'To put it another way, you provide, when you are well, a service that will be available if and when you fall ill. It is therefore an act of collective goodwill and public enterprise and not a commodity privately bought and sold. It takes away a whole segment of private enterprise and transfers it to the field of public administration, where it joins company with the preventative services and the rest of the communal agencies, by means of which the new society is being gradually articulated. . . .

'Danger of abuse in the Health Service is always at the point where private commercialism impinges on the Service. . . . Does it therefore follow that the solution is to abandon the field to commercialism? Of course not. The solution is to decrease the dependence on private enterprise. . . .

'A free health Service is a triumphant example of the superiority of collective action and the public initiative applied to a segment of society where commercial principles are seen at their worst.'

Document 3

Extract from Arthur Seldon's *Wither the Welfare State* (1981) in which he sets out the case against state welfare and in favour of markets. (Reproduced with the permission of the Institute of Economic Affairs.)

THE FLAWS OF THE WELFARE STATE AND THE FLAWS OF THE POLITICAL STATE

'The political state has seven deadly sins and the welfare state displays all of them.

'*First*, it is based on ignorance of the preferences of consumers – parents, patients, home-occupiers, pensioners – because it has no machinery for gathering information from individuals. . . .

'*Second*, ignorance provokes inefficiency. . . .

'*Third*, the welfare state replaced choice for consumers between competing suppliers by monopoly from which there is no escape, except at a cost that the rich can bear better than the poor. . . .

'*Fourth*, the welfare state, contrary to the claims of its sponsors, becomes unjust, inequitable, unrepresentative, unaccountable and inegalitarian. . . .

'*Fifth*, the welfare state creates social conflict because the distribution of its benefits is decided by activists elected by majorities – or even minorities – in both national and local government. . . . Parties are organised, managed and directed by the politically-inclined, the politically active, the politically adroit, the politically artful. But most people are not, least of all the ordinary people, the working class. In the state they lose to the few who are, who can argue their way into, or buy homes near, the best state schools. In the market the ordinary people are, or can be made, equal in status as consumers. . . .

'*Sixth*, the welfare state rests on coercion. It empowers majorities to coerce minorities, groups and individuals. . . .

'*Seventh*, the disarming description "welfare" must not be allowed to conceal the truth that the welfare state harbours the same opportunities and incitements to abuse and even corruption as the non-welfare state. . . . A man or woman does not become a saint by being appointed a "public" official . . . the inescapable conclusion [is] that the welfare state, national and local, must be tainted or riddled with corruption. . . . The power-hungry, the bureaucrat, the technocrat, the ideologue and the autocrat find openings in all systems. . . . In the market the abuses are worst where there is a monopoly. But monopoly in the market is not endemic: it can be disciplined by changes in supply and demand, or limited by law. In the state, monopoly is the very essence.

'*Eighth* . . . the welfare state will use secrecy to avoid being judged. For its operators are judges and juries in their own cause. . . .

'We cannot depend upon a government of any party to liquidate the welfare state as an act of patriotism or in response to public preferences. In the end it will be market forces that will make the welfare state yield to private choice and technical advance.'

Document 4

Extract from the Conservative Party Manifesto, General Election 1987, *The Next Move Forward*, London, The Conservative Party.

'WIDER OWNERSHIP AND GREATER OPPORTUNITY

'Conservatives aim to extend as widely as possible the opportunity to own property and build up capital, to exercise real choice in education, and to develop economic independence and security.

'Our goal is a capital-owning democracy of people and families who exercise power over their own lives in the most direct way. *They* would take the important decisions – as tenants, home-owners, parents, employees, and trade unionists – rather than having them taken for them.

'. . . What the Conservative Government *has* done is to make it easier for people to acquire independence for themselves:

'– by introducing the right to buy council houses;
'– by returning nationalised industries to the people in ways that encourage the widest possible spread of ownership;
'– by making it easier to buy shares in British industry.

'. . . There has been a surge of home-ownership, share-ownership and self-reliance.

'. . . In this way the scope of individual responsibility is widened, the family is strengthened, and voluntary bodies flourish. State power is checked and opportunities are spread throughout society.

'BETTER HOUSING FOR ALL

'Home ownership

'Nowhere has the spread of ownership been more significant than in housing. Buying their own home is the first step most people take towards building up capital to hand down to their children and grandchildren. It gives people a stake in society – something to conserve. It is the foundation stone of a capital-owning democracy.

'. . . Home-ownership has been the great success story of housing policy in the last eight years. One million council tenants have become home-owners and another one and a half million more families have become home-owners for the first time.

'Two out of every three homes are now owned by the people who live in them. This is a very high proportion, one of the largest in the world. *We are determined to make it larger still.*

'. . . After eight years of Conservative Government, Britain is now at the forefront of a world-wide revolution in extending ownership.

'. . . This is the first stage of a profound and progressive social transformation – popular capitalism. Owning a direct stake in industry not only enhances personal independence; it also gives a heightened sense of involvement and pride in British business.

'In the Next Parliament

'. . . We will privatise more state industries in ways that increase share-ownership, both for the employees and for the public at large.

'Raising Standards in Education

'Parents want schools to provide their children with the knowledge, training and character that will fit them for today's world. They want them to be taught basic educational skills. They want schools that will encourage moral values; honesty, hard work and responsibility. And they should have the right to choose those schools which do these things for their children.

'Raising Standards in our Schools

'Four Major Reforms
'First, we will establish a National Core Curriculum.

'. . . Second, within five years governing bodies and head teachers of all secondary schools and many primary schools will be given control over their own budgets.

'. . . Third, we will increase parental choice.

'. . . We will ensure that Local Education Authorities (LEAs) set school budgets in line with the number of pupils who will be attending each school.

'. . . We will support the co-existence of a variety of schools – comprehensive, grammar, secondary modern, voluntary controlled and aided, independent, sixth form and tertiary colleges all of which will give parents greater choice and lead to higher standards.

'We will establish a pilot network of City Technology Colleges.

'We will expand the Assisted Places Scheme to 35,000.

'. . . We will allow state schools to opt out of LEA control.'

Document 5

Extract from a speech made by the Secretary of State for Health, Virginia Bottomley to the Harvard Medical School, *Lessons, Challenges and Opportunities of Health Reform*, 31 May 1995. (Reproduced with the permission of the Controller of Her Majesty's Stationery Office © Crown Copyright.)

'The 1991 reforms left unchanged the aspects of the NHS which constitute its core ethos and values: universal access, treatment on the basis of clinical need rather than ability to pay, and financing from general taxation. They have broken with the past, divesting the NHS of its old centralising strait-jacket, and introducing flexibility and diversity to make a national service more locally responsive.

'After 40 years the NHS had begun to show its age. The centralised "command and control" system that had been installed in the 1940s was proving increasingly stifling and bureaucratic. . . .

'The old NHS was seen as increasingly unresponsive to patients. The patients who thronged its doors behaved like – and were often treated as – grateful supplicants rather than empowered consumers. . . .

'The changes have led to a more decentralised service with greater flexibility and responsiveness to the needs of patients and underpinned by more and better information about benefits and costs. Local pay is a further logical extension of this process, giving employers in Trusts control over what is 70 per cent of their costs.

'Power has passed from planners in the Department of Health or in regional health authorities to staff working closest to patients. The point about fundholding is that it gives doctors muscle in the system by giving them a budget they control. . . . The result has been to unlock the potential which exists among individuals for innovation and initiative.

'. . . Maintaining this progress is no easy task as the public's expectations and their demands on finite resources grow ever greater.

'Pressures on the NHS – and all health care systems – are going to continue. But a consensus is beginning to be established that we have the right structures in place and the issue is to realise the potential they offer and meet the challenges ahead.'

Document 6

Extract from a speech by Secretary of State for Health, Stephen Dorrell, to the Royal College of Physicians in London, in which the Minister set out the Government's case for the Private Finance Initiative, November 1995. (Reproduced with the permission of the Controller of Her Majesty's Stationery Office © Crown Copyright.)

'PFI contracts give the private sector a completely different incentive. The consortium, which often includes a construction company, will continue to be responsible for managing the facility in use. In both the design and construction phase they therefore have a clear incentive to produce a facility which has a low full life cost, rather than a low construction cost. It is an important distinction, which will work to the long-term benefit of the NHS.

'The fact that the private sector will also take responsibility for generating income from outside the NHS has also allowed a number of schemes to include retail units, leisure centres, and other developments such as office buildings or media parks. These proposals have allowed fuller and more economic use of hospital sites with the result that capital assets that have hitherto been under used will now be used to the full for the benefit of patients of the NHS.

'Perhaps most important of all, it demonstrates a final abandonment of a dogmatic assertion that public and private sector must be kept totally separate. The PFI allows the private sector the opportunity to use its skills to modernise NHS facilities where it can demonstrate good value. And it allows the NHS to concentrate its resources, both financial and human, on its central priority – the development of high-quality clinical care.

'It puts patients before politics; that is why I believe that it should command the support of all those who wish the NHS well.'

Document 7

Extract from the 10th Report of the Social Security Advisory Committee 1995, London, HMSO. (Reproduced with the permission of the Controller of Her Majesty's Stationery Office on behalf of Parliament © Parliamentary Copyright.)

'STATE BENEFITS AND PRIVATE PROVISION

'In the case of incapacity, disability and unemployment, we could see little scope for developing private provision to an extent which would impact on state benefits. There is clearly a market for private insurance against these contingencies and it will doubtless continue to develop, but coverage may be prohibitively expensive for those most at risk of needing to draw on it. For some people, such as those disabled from childhood and unable to work, private insurance is unlikely ever to be an option.

'Universal coverage regardless of risk is the great strength of the state scheme and unless this could be replicated by the insurance industry, at affordable cost, we could see little prospect of private provision supplanting state benefits for the vast majority of the population, and for high risk, vulnerable groups in particular.

'One area where the private sector has already assumed an important and growing role is in the field of provision for retirement. Increasing levels of private income, at present mainly from occupational pensions, are being enjoyed by many recently retired people, and it is clear that occupational and personal pensions are set to continue to form a growing part of income in retirement, although we considered that the growth in part-time work and other changes in patterns of employment may cause the rate of expansion to be checked. At the same time, the basic state retirement pension, on its own, is now significantly lower than income support. Prices indexation of the basic pension since 1980 has resulted in a steady decline in its value relative to earnings. If current policies continue, its value to future generations will be minimal.

'. . . Our principal concern is for the many people – those with low life-time earnings (especially women), the long-term unemployed and others with interrupted work patterns, and sick and disabled people – who are unable to benefit from the expansion in private provision for retirement. There will clearly be a continuing need for state provision for an adequate income during retirement for a very significant number of people, and we stressed the value of the contributory state pension as an inter-generational contract – a fundamental commitment on the part of the whole community to ensure a minimum income for those who have retired. We do not believe that it would be acceptable to abandon the contributory contract for a pension based solely on means.

'We considered that mortgage insurance was another area where private provision might assume greater importance in future. We noted that the cover offered by such insurance was often very limited and that, in practice, existing borrowers found it difficult to obtain. But we suggested that, given the development of suitable packages (perhaps with mortgagors taking a pooled risk approach), greater reliance on the private sector might be possible. At the time of writing, the Government has already imposed a limit of £125,000 on loans for which help would be given under income support. We took the view that alternative forms of insurance should be available and in place before any further reduction in state support. However, we saw a continuing need for state help with mortgage costs for people who are long-term unemployed, sick or disabled, lone parents and pensioners. It appeared to us to be extremely unlikely that private mortgage insurance could ever be developed to provide a long-term cover required by people in these circumstances.

'Since the publication of our paper, the Government has further restricted the help available to home owners under the income support scheme.'

Document 8

Extracts from three 1996 speeches by Secretary of State for Education and Employment, Gillian Sheppard, in which she summarised the outcomes of Conservative education policies to date, and planned further reforms for the future. (Reproduced with the permission of the Controller of Her Majesty's Stationery Office © Crown Copyright.)

Document 8(a) Extract from speech to National Children's Bureau Conference, *The Future Shape of Early Years Services*, February 1996.

'Last month, as you will know, I introduced the Government's Bill to expand the education of under 5s. . . . I admit to being a little disappointed by the negative reaction the nursery education initiative has received in some quarters. It is not every day that government commits itself unequivocally to expansion of a service; puts up substantial new money to make it happen; consults on all the main details; and promises a new structure for ensuring quality. On top of that, we aim to extend parental choice as much as possible, and draw on the strengths of a varied system. . . .

'Let me make the Government's position perfectly clear. We want to make available to all young children the personal, social and educational benefits that arise from a significant period of good pre-school education. We want to do so in a way that maximises choice for parents, the people who are best placed to judge their children's needs. I recognise that the providers of nursery education have needs too, but in my view they cannot be put ahead of the needs of parents and their children.

'I see nothing objectionable or harmful in those objectives, or in the way we propose to achieve them. Parents will surely applaud the commitment to new places, to quality and to choice. Providers should welcome the injection of additional resources, the opportunity to expand, the stimulus to raise standards. Local authorities and maintained schools will gain resources, not lose them, if their nursery education is attractive to parents. Good private and voluntary providers can take their places alongside the maintained sector as partners of equal standing. . . .

'Perhaps because educational vouchers as an instrument of parental choice are a new concept in Britain, or perhaps just to make mischief, myths have been peddled about the effects of the scheme. . . . There has been a lot of wild talk about the damaging effects of competition. It may well be in the interest of both the maintained and the private and voluntary sectors to look at the possibility of forging partnerships. But, there is nothing wrong in parents exercising choice and this is at the centre, the real essence, of the scheme.

'. . . Key words are choice, diversity and quality. Vouchers are worrying some people, no doubt. But they need not. If providers are giving parents what they want, vouchers can only reinforce that. The quality assurance regime will ensure that we do not simply have an expansion of places, but places of good quality. I firmly believe the new nursery education scheme will be a major force for raising educational standards and advancing parental choice.'

Document 8(b) Extract from speech made in London on the first anniversary of the Government's *Improving Schools* programme, June 1996.

'Much has changed for the better in recent years:

'– We have introduced the National Curriculum with testing and assessment of all 7-, 11- and 14-year-olds in English, mathematics and science. Results for 11-year-olds will be published in performance tables like the GCSE results.
'– We have reinforced parent power by publishing information on schools and linking funding to pupil numbers so that schools have incentives to offer what parents want. We have let schools opt out and become grant-maintained,

encouraged specialisation in particular subjects, and offered assisted places in good independent schools to over 75,000 children since 1981.
'– We are inspecting all schools within a four-year cycle. All schools must have action plans. Failing schools must improve, or close within two years.

'At the end of June there will be a major White Paper on schools. It will focus on extending self-government, choice and diversity.

'We have developed local management of schools, giving local authority schools power to decide how to spend their budgets.

'The White Paper will extend local management. Local authorities will have to pass on more of the available funds to schools.

'We will also give grant-maintained schools more power to decide their future development and to take on services which local authorities currently provide. This will include more freedom to select children by ability or by aptitude for particular subjects.

'We want parents to be able to choose – from a range of good schools – the education that best suits their children.

'We want a spectrum of schools reflecting the varied talents and needs of our children. Grammar and other selective schools are an essential part of that.

'The White Paper on schools will propose extending opportunities for selection:

'– we will make it easier for schools to select pupils by ability or aptitude – including opting for full grammar school status;
'– we will allow schools to select more of their pupils without seeking central approval.

'The White Paper will also encourage more schools to specialise in particular subjects.

'High standards of teaching and learning require classrooms to be orderly places. . . . The next step will be legislation in the Autumn to bolster schools' authority in dealing with discipline problems. This will:

'– allow schools to detain pupils after school, irrespective of parents' consent;
'– give schools flexibility to suspend pupils temporarily for up to 45 days.

'We are also looking at:

'– changes to the arrangements for appeals against exclusion;
'– allowing oversubscribed schools to insist on home-school contracts as a condition for admission;
'– limiting choice of school for pupils excluded more than once;
'– whether we can find ways to bring penalties to bear more effectively on truants and their parents.

'The Assisted Places Scheme, established in 1981, allows able children from less well-off families to benefit from a first rate education at independent schools. . . .

'In taking forward this agenda we will make sure we keep a focus on basic skills.

'I have asked SCAA for advice on baseline assessment as the starting point for measuring progress in the early years. The revised national curriculum has a sharper focus on English and maths, and within maths on number. We have introduced a calculator-free test for 11-year-olds this year, and will do the same for 14-year-olds from next year. We are considering a mental arithmetic test for 11- and 14-year-olds.'

Document 8(c) Extract from speech on the second reading of the Government's 1996 *Education Bill*, November 1996.

'One of the great strengths of this Government has been to provide and promote choice and diversity. This Bill will enable us to go further. We want to give schools greater freedom to introduce or extend selection and specialisation.

'We are not in the business of imposing two types of schools, we welcome all types. The only uniformity we insist on is that they should all provide a good education. We would like to see more grammar schools if that is what parents want.

'GM status gives schools the sense that they are responsible for what they do. It unlocks energy, initiative and commitment. In addition to the power to select more of their pupils the Bill also enables GM schools to add nursery classes, sixth forms and boarding facilities and to expand their capacity by up to 50 per cent without central approval.

'The Government's over-riding objective in education is to raise standards in schools. All of the measures in the Bill have that one aim in mind. The selection and deregulation measures will help create a pattern of schools in which each can develop its own strengths. The discipline measures will help create an environment within schools in which good teaching and learning can take place. But the Bill also targets some specific areas for action to raise standards.

'Choice and diversity for parents. Clear expectations of pupils. Accountability with freedom for schools. These are the principles we have made our own and applied consistently. Through this Bill we shall continue to apply them for the benefit of all the children of this country.'

Document 9

Press release from the Department of Social Security, announcing Peter Lilley's intention to privatise the delivery of social security benefits. (Reproduced with the permission of the Controller of Her Majesty's Stationery Office © Crown Copyright.)

'19 July 1996

'PETER LILLEY ANNOUNCES NEW INITIATIVES UNDER THE CHANGE PROGRAMME

'Peter Lilley, Secretary of State for Social Security, today announced further private sector involvement in the Department's drive to improve the delivery of benefits.

'In answer to a parliamentary question from Mrs Marion Roe(Broxbourne), Mr Lilley said:

"In February, I launched the Change Programme to achieve a step change in the effectiveness of the Department of Social Security and all its Agencies. It will involve streamlining benefit processes, introducing new information technology and greater involvement of the private sector.

"I have today approved three initiatives involving greater collaboration with the private sector as the next stage of the Department's drive to review and improve the delivery of social security.

"The first initiative will involve an invitation to the private sector to submit proposals for taking over the operation of the Child Benefit Centre in Washington, Tyne and Wear. This will involve the administration of Child Benefit, One Parent Benefit and Guardians Allowance. The intention is that staff working in these areas will be taken on by the appointed contractor.

"The second initiative will involve three private companies – or consortia – appointed following open competition to work in conjunction with the Benefits Agency in running benefit delivery in three of its thirteen areas (Yorkshire, West Country and East London & Anglia Area Directorates) for twelve months.

"All three companies will assist the Benefits Agency with the development of new business processes and information technology. They will be invited during the twelve month period to submit proposals for any elements of the Agency's business which could be run differently, including the possibility of further parts of the operation being run by the private sector.

"The third initiative is to launch the procurement process for an Information Systems/Information Technology strategy to enable greater sharing of data between benefit systems, working closely with the private sector to provide the most up to date technologies, expertise and funding.

"These initiatives are designed to improve the administration of the benefit system. They will not change any individual's benefit entitlement."'

Document 10

Contrasting views of two Secretaries of State, in relation to social services, 1997 and 1998. (Reproduced with the permission of the Controller of Her Majesty's Stationery Office © Crown Copyright.)

Document 10(a) is an extract from a press release announcing the Conservative White Paper *Social Services: Achievement and Challenge*, March 1997.

Document 10(b) is an extract from the Labour White Paper *Modernising Social Services, Promoting Independence, Improving Protection, Raising Standards*, published in November 1998.

Document 10(A)

'Radical plans to reform the delivery and structure of social services were un-veiled today in a White Paper launched by Health Secretary Stephen Dorrell.

'The White Paper – *Social Services: Achievement and Challenge* – introduces a purchaser–provider split in the delivery of care, fresh opportunities for the independent sector, new measures to bring greater value for money. . . .

'A Social Services Reform Bill would require councils to concentrate on care assessment and commissioning, leaving the provision of residential care for adults to the independent sector. Councils could only provide residential care and home helps if independent providers were unable to meet local needs.

'The White Paper says that the three functions of social services – assessing and commissioning care; providing care; and regulation of care services – should be separated clearly from each other.

'Stephen Dorrell said:

"The changes proposed in the White Paper reflect the Government's view that in a modern society, the principal responsibility for meeting social care needs rests on the individual citizen planning to meet their own needs and responding to the needs of their family and their neighbours. The role of statut-ory social services is to act as a support to those, including carers, who are meeting social care needs in these ways."'

Document 10(B)

'November 1998 Cm 4169

'1.1 Social services are for all of us. At any one time up to one and a half million people in England rely on their help. And all of us are likely at some point in our lives to need to turn to social services for support, whether on our own behalf or for a family member. . . .'

'1.2 We all depend on good social services to be there at such times of crisis, to help in making the right decisions and working out what needs to be done. And more widely, we all benefit if social services are providing good, effective ser-vices to those who need them. . . .'

'1.3 Social services, therefore, do not just support a small number of "social casualties"; they are an important part of the fabric of a caring society. It is a concern for everyone that social services should be providing the best possible service.'

'1.7 The proposals in the White Paper look to the future, to the creation of modern social services. The last Government's devotion to privatisation of care provision put dogma before users' interests, and threatened a fragmentation of vital services. But it is also true that the near-monopoly local authority provision that used to be a feature of social care led to a "one size fits all" approach where users were expected to accommodate themselves to the services that existed.

Our third way for social care moves the focus away from who provides the care, and places it firmly on the quality of services experienced by, and outcomes achieved for, individuals and their carers and families.'

'2.1 Social services for adults are right at the heart of the welfare state.'

'2.25 Many people feel that the care system is not fair. There are variations in who gets what services, inconsistencies in what types of provision are available in different parts of the country, and differences in how charging works.'

'2.29 The differences in these discretionary charges can be considerable. The amount that authorities recover in charges – as a percentage of their spending on these services – varies from 4 per cent to 28 per cent. And the charging systems differ enormously from one council to another. For instance, one council might charge a standard hourly rate which everyone – whatever their income – pays, so that the amount paid depends on the amount of care received. Whereas another council might operate a sliding scale of charges according to income, regardless of how much care is received. . . .'

'2.30 It has always been the case that the user has been expected to contribute to the cost of some services, particularly residential care, according to an assessment of income. However, there are strong criticisms of the system, both in terms of the fairness of the national charging system for residential care, and in terms of the variation, from one part of the country to another, of the discretionary charges for services in the community.'

'2.37 There must be greater transparency and fairness in the contribution that people are asked to make towards their social care. We are committed to finding a way to fund long term care which is fair and affordable for the individual and the taxpayer.'

'2.40 The Government believes that the scale of variation in the discretionary charging system, including the difference in how income is assessed, is unacceptable. We will consider how to improve the system in the light of both the Royal Commission's report and the Audit Commission survey.'

'7.23 Best value must be secured in all social services, whether provided in-house or contracted out to the voluntary or private sector. This Government does not take an ideological approach to this issue, and has no preconception about whether the public or the voluntary or private sector should be the preferred providers. These decisions should be based entirely on judgements about best value and optimum outcomes for individual users, and authorities must be able to demonstrate that their arrangements are delivering this.'

'7.24 By the same token, we are keen to remove any distorting effects there are in the current system for authorities to use one sector over the other, and keen to give councils as much flexibility as possible in making effective use of public money available for care.'

Document 11

Extracts from the Prime Minister's speech on 2 June 1997, at the Aylesbury estate, Southwark. (Reproduced with the permission of the Controller of Her Majesty's Stationery Office © Crown Copyright.)

'THE WILL TO WIN

'I have chosen this housing estate to deliver my first speech as Prime Minister for a very simple reason. For 18 years, the poorest people in our country have been forgotten by government. They have been left out of growing prosperity, told that they were not needed, ignored by the Government except for the purpose of blaming them. I want that to change. There will be no forgotten people in the Britain I want to build.

'We need to act in a new way because fatalism, and not just poverty, is the problem we face, the dead weight of low expectations, the crushing belief that things cannot get better. I want to give people back the will to win again. This will to win is what drives a country, the belief that expectations can be fulfilled and ambitions realised.

'But that cannot be done without a radical shift in our values and attitudes. . . .

'The 1960s were the decade of "anything goes". The 1980s were a time of "who cares?". The next decade will be defined by a simple idea; "we are all in this together". It will be about how to recreate the bonds of civic society and community in a way compatible with the far more individualistic nature of modern, economic, social and cultural life. . . .

'But this new alliance of interests to build on "one nation Britain" can only be done on the basis of a new bargain between us all as members of society.

'We should reject the rootless morality whose symptom is a false choice between bleeding hearts and couldn't care less, when what we need is one grounded in the core of British values, the sense of fairness and a balance between rights and duties.

'The basis of this modern civic society is an ethic of mutual responsibility or duty. It is something for something. A society where we play by the rules. You only take out if you put in. That's the bargain.

'In concrete terms that means:

'• Reforming welfare so that government helps people to help themselves and provides for those who can't, rather than trying to do it all through government.
'• Where opportunities are given, for example to young people, for real jobs and skills, there should be a reciprocal duty on them to take them up.
'• We should encourage people like single mothers who are anxious to work but unable to, to get back into the labour market. This is empowerment not punishment.

'• We should root out educational failure, because it is the greatest inhibition to correcting poverty.
'• We should enforce a new code of laws that crack down on crime and other antisocial behaviour.
'• We should attack discrimination in all its forms.
'• We should engage the interest and commitment of the whole of the community to tackle the desperate need for urban regeneration.
'• Government should commit itself to using whatever means is the best to play its part without outdated dogma of left or right to hold it back.

'. . . Earlier this century leaders faced the challenge of creating a welfare state that could provide security for the new working class. Today the greatest challenge of any democratic government is to refashion our institutions to bring this new workless class back into society and into useful work, and to bring back the will to win.

'. . . What unites these policies is the idea that work is the best form of welfare – the best way of funding people's needs, and the best way of giving them a stake in society. They will help the under-25s who are the first generation since the war to expect their standard of living to be worse than their parents.

'To reverse the slide towards a divided nation, we also need to tap a wider ethic of responsibility. The making of one nation is not just a job for government. It is a task for everyone, a responsibility that applies as much at the top of society as at the bottom.

'Unless Government is pragmatic and rigorous about what does and does not work, it will not spend money wisely or gain the trust of the public. The last Government did little serious evaluation of its policies for poverty, and didn't even know how many people had been on welfare for 10 or 20 years. Its policies were driven by dogma, not by common sense.

'Our approach will be different. We will find out what works, and we will support the successes and stop the failures. We will back anyone – from a multinational company to a community association – if they can deliver the goods. . . . We will, in short, govern in a different way. In the 1960s people thought government was always the solution. In the 1980s people said government was the problem. In the 1990s, we know that we cannot solve the problems of the workless class without government, but that government itself must change if it is to be part of the solution not the problem.

'. . . There already is a sense of hope and optimism in the country. People believe that there are new options, new possibilities. And I want everyone to be part of them.

'That is a new Government with a new sense of purpose. A Government that believes in giving everyone the chance to succeed and get on in life. It is a Government that has a will to win. To those who have lost hope over the last 18 years, I offer them a fresh start. The best thing any Government can offer is hope, and that is what I bring today.'

Document 12

Extracts from a speech made by the Secretary of State for Education, David Blunkett, to the Technology Colleges Trust, 5 November 1997.

'Diversity and Specialism will Boost Standards

'Business has provided over £3 million extra sponsorship for specialist schools in the last six months – which will help to promote the Government's aims of diversity and excellence in secondary education', Education and Employment Secretary David Blunkett said today. Total sponsorship for specialist schools in 1998/99 is expected to be over £9 million.

'Setting out his commitment to expanding specialist schools – which cover technology, language, arts and sports – from just under 260 at present to over 300 from next September at the Annual Lecture of the Technology Colleges Trust at the Banqueting House in Whitehall, Mr Blunkett said:

"Specialist schools are at the heart of my vision – and that of the new Government – of an education system where education caters for the individual strengths of children rather than assuming a bland sameness for all.

"Some people were surprised that the Government wanted to continue the specialist schools programme. They do not understand the philosophy of the new Government. We welcomed this great opportunity to further the causes of school improvement and school diversity. By building on the excellent work already in place and broadening the reach of the programme we intend to ensure it is open to as many children as possible – both those attending specialist schools and those in neighbouring schools enjoying their facilities.

"As we approach the millennium, we must have more specialist schools which offer diversity within a single campus. We must allow children to play to their individual strengths and aptitudes – those who want to see sameness for all are betraying our children. We must move from an education system which caters for the producers to one which puts the needs of the consumers – pupils and their parents – at the heart of its approach.

"Comprehensive education must modernise. It cannot forever be stuck in the past – what some might see as a sixties time warp. High and improving standards, setting by subject ability and the ability to foster specialist talents must all be part of the way forward. These are all a key part of the programme set out in our Excellence in Schools consultation paper – on which we have received a substantial and positive response.

"One of the ways we will do this is to give specialist schools a new role from next September in providing masterclasses for gifted children from neighbouring primary schools. We are still working on the details but we hope to see the role extended to secondary schools later on.

"The subject area focus of specialist schools is an excellent basis for development planning to bring about whole school improvement. The disciplines of planning, target setting and monitoring performance spread the advantages across the school. Our new emphasis on a community approach will spread the resource advantages well beyond the boundaries of the specialist schools themselves. They will share facilities and expertise with local schools. That means nearby secondary schools as well as feeder primary schools. And developments in Information and Communications Technology blur the definition of nearby schools, spreading the net of possibilities.

"We want inclusiveness in education. Inclusive in access to the opportunities and inclusive in the opportunities for partnership. The right to a good education is above politics. And good ideas about education have a right to stand outside politics. I am delighted to build on the specialist school policy. And I am pleased we have had a marvellous private sector response to our new community approach.

"Through the Technology Colleges Trust well over £3 million has been raised from major companies and foundations since we relaunched the programme under the banner Education Partnerships for the 21st century. . . . The private sector partnership, in getting involved with schools even more than in giving money, is a vital part of this inclusive programme and I am pleased by the response.

". . . In his pre-election speech in Birmingham the Prime Minister said he was looking to expand the programme to 450 schools by the year 2001. . . . I am determined to find funding from existing resources for expansion of the specialist schools programme.

"My immediate aim is to increase the number of schools from the current 258 to over 300 by next September. That will mean nearly 400,000 secondary school pupils will be attending specialist schools – and hundreds of thousands more will be benefiting from partnerships through a 'family of schools' approach." '

Document 13

Extracts from a speech by Alistair Darling, Secretary of State for Social Security, Institute of Public Policy Research, *Modernising the Welfare State for the Next Millennium*, September 1998. (Reproduced with the permission of the Controller of Her Majesty's Stationery Office © Crown Copyright.)

'Today, too much of what is done by the welfare state is out of date, or done in an out of date way. And the result is some people are poorer than they need be, others dependent on benefit when they need not be, and still others neglected when they need not be.

'. . . Economic, social and demographic change has occurred on a massive scale. These changes must influence how we reform welfare. Something else has changed too – the degree to which people make provision for themselves. That provision isn't and shouldn't be a monopoly of the public sector. Far from it. Increasingly people look to both the public and private sector, together with the voluntary sector, to work together. Pensions are provided both by the state and by employers and insurance companies. In 1953, only 28 per cent of employees were in an occupational pension scheme. Now over two-thirds of contributing employees are in either an occupational or personal pension. Increased pension provision over and above government support has been a key factor behind rising general pensioner incomes. Insurance against death, sickness and disability has also grown in importance. In 1995, two-thirds of households had some type of insurance, providing for an average lump sum cover of £12,000. And almost 1½ million people have taken out insurance policies for incapacity.

'So we need to build on that partnership between public and private provision – another principle from the Green Paper. State spending should be concentrated where it is needed most – families in need, pensioners on low incomes, the severely disabled for whom work is not a realistic prospect. In modernising the welfare state, we need to adapt and respond to the major social and economic changes we face in the future. In doing so, we must ensure that spending meets our priorities. Thus the pensioner guarantee or help for getting people into work – the New Deal.

'And it isn't a choice between "means-testing" on the one hand and a "contributory" system on the other. That is a false dichotomy. Contributory benefits have rarely been operated without any form of conditionality. Other benefits have been designed to help those with extra costs: winter fuel payments or help focused on children through child benefit. What we need is a sensible mixed economy where people have the encouragement and support to contribute when they can, so that public and private provision increasingly work together – pensions for example. Where the post-war pioneers thought of state provision as an alternative to private provision, today we need a partnership between public and private sectors.

'And the role of the welfare state has to change too. Where the current welfare state is passive, reacting to events, the new welfare state must be active. Where too often the focus has been only on cash benefits, in the future it must be about services as well. As the Green Paper sets out, the new welfare state should help and encourage people of working age to work where they are capable of doing so.

'. . . The Green Paper sets out a clear philosophy for the welfare state. 'Work for those who can, security for those who cannot' is the foundation of our programme. It has received overwhelming support.

'. . . We need to move away from the idea that worklessness must be idleness. In the next century we should be aiming for a system that ensures that if people who can work are not in work they should be actively preparing or looking for work. And the New Deals show how the modern welfare state can do that.

'. . . Our objective is to help people prepare for and get work as well as making work pay. That is why we are determined to use every opportunity to help those who can work to do so. The test must be one of capacity not incapacity. We will reform the gateways to the benefit system so that everyone has the best possible advice. Everyone who is able to do so should have the opportunity to work. They have a right to expect that help. And a responsibility to take up that help. By cutting the bills of economic failure we can devote more resources to our priorities.

'. . . As we said in the Green Paper, we also want to shift the focus from what people can't do to what they can. In some cases Incapacity Benefit writes off as unfit for work people who might, with some assistance, be able to return to work.

'. . . Of course, there are other areas in need of reform too. Over the longer term it cannot make sense to have a system in which tenants on benefit have little interest in the rent. At present, provided it meets local limits, Housing Benefit will meet it in full.

'We want to build a system which is less prone to abuse or fraud; which does less damage to work incentives and makes more sense in economic terms.

'. . . And we want to build new partnerships with the private sector so mortgage payment protection insurance plays a more effective role alongside the state's support in helping home-owners who get into difficulty . . . whereas the pioneers of the welfare state saw the choice as being between public provision or private provision, that is not the case today. Partnership in provision will continue to grow.

'Social security no longer fits today's world, still less the world of the next millennium. We were elected to reform and modernise the welfare state. We have an ambitious programme for reform based on the principles in the Green Paper. We were elected to deliver and deliver it we will.'

Document 14

Extract from the Select Committee on Public Accounts, Sixty-First Report *Getting Value for Money in Privatisations*, September 1998. (Reproduced with the permission of the Controller of Her Majesty's Stationery Office © Parliamentary Copyright.)

'For nearly 20 years the United Kingdom has led the world in the privatisation of state-owned businesses. During that time over 150 United Kingdom businesses have been privatised, ranging from major undertakings worth billions of pounds to small loss-making enterprises. In the process, the proportion of Gross Domestic Product accounted for by state-owned businesses has fallen from 11 per cent to 2 per cent.

'These privatisations have shared a number of overall objectives, including improving the efficiency of the business concerned, promoting the development of the market economy, reducing state debt and increasing state revenues. Government departments have acknowledged throughout that, in the interests of the taxpayer, and having regard to the particular objectives of the sale, they have a duty to do all they can to maximise the proceeds from each sale. Moreover, the yield from these sales has been considerable, £90 billion (at current prices) so far. Departments have, in many cases, become increasingly expert in their conduct of sales, stimulating external advisers and the markets to accept an increasingly sophisticated range of sales techniques aimed at ensuring that the taxpayer gets as good a deal as possible.

'In studying and reporting on these sales, the Committee and its predecessors have, however, noted a number of instances, often recurring, in which for a variety of reasons departments have failed to maximise proceeds, or have fallen short of the care which they are expected to exercise in disposing of public assets. It is the invariable practice of the Committee of Public Accounts not to make any judgements about the rights or wrongs of the policy of privatisations *per se* but, given that a policy has been pursued, we do examine the effectiveness, efficiency and value for money achieved in the operation of that policy. The purpose of this report is to draw attention both to the types of cases in which departments could have achieved a better result for the taxpayer, and cases where, by contrast, as a result of careful planning and a preparedness to innovate, they have achieved good value for money.

'Part 1 of this report sets out key lessons on which we and our predecessors have reported, including important general issues relating to sale objectives, restructuring, valuations, timing, and the skills required by vendor departments. We also underline important lessons relating to the two main privatisation methods used in the United Kingdom: first, flotations and share sales; and second, trade sales, that is the sale of the state-owned business directly to another business or to its management and/or employees.

'. . . Some of these issues, for example the appointment of advisers through competition, raise important questions of propriety. Most, however, are about the difficult choices departments face in marketing business opportunities while protecting the taxpayers' interests. They have to take their decisions confronted by uncertainty and it is not for us, with the benefit of hindsight, to understate the challenges they face. We recognise that they have to exercise judgement. Nevertheless, it should be judgement well grounded in experience and expertise.

'The privatisation of state-owned enterprises is, of course, only one aspect of the ways in which the public and private sectors are working together. The Government have announced a programme of public–private partnerships in which sales of shareholdings in state-owned businesses are likely to feature and, as the public sector continues to develop its role of purchaser as well as provider of public services, new forms of relationships are developing, including further projects under the private finance initiative, joint ventures, the disposal of surplus assets, and the increasingly commercial use of assets remaining in state ownership. We believe that the lessons set out in this report will remain of value to departments as they seek to get the best possible deal for the taxpayers.'

Document 15

Secretary of State for Health, Frank Dobson, welcomes the Acheson *Report into Inequalities in Health*, and sets out the Government's approach to public health improvement, November 1998. (Reproduced with the permission of the Controller of Her Majesty's Stationery Office © Parliamentary Copyright.)

'The whole Government, led from the top by the Prime Minister, is committed to the greatest ever reduction in health inequalities.

'In July 1997, shortly after taking office, I invited Sir Donald Acheson to conduct an inquiry into health inequalities in Britain. That was because I was determined to make an early start on our mission to reduce inequalities in health as part of our overall programme to improve the health of the nation. Today I welcome his report. It is a further stage in our unprecedented commitment to tackle inequalities in health.

'No previous Government has ever set itself such ambitious targets. But we are confident we can succeed. That's because the whole of the Government is taking action. Led by the Prime Minister, all the Cabinet are working together to tackle the things that make people ill.

'Poverty is a principal source of ill-health. Poor people are ill more often and die sooner. Our tax and benefit changes, the Working Families Tax Credit and the minimum wage mean that work will pay a guaranteed minimum of £190 a week for a family. That will guarantee a minimum income of at least £5.50 an hour for a lone parent in work with one child and £6.37 for an adult with two children.

'A poor start in life is bad for your health. Our £540 million Sure Start programme will give young children and their parents the child care and support they need, so that every child in our country gets the best start in life.

'A decent education sets you up for better health in later life. As part of our work to drive up standards in all schools, earlier this month we announced an extra £250 million aimed at children who are disaffected with school or society at large.

'Being old and cold in winter because you haven't the money to buy yourself warm clothes and good food – or are afraid to turn on the fire – is bad for your health. So our £2.5 billion pensions boost to ensure that poorest pensioners are the biggest winners, with a guaranteed minimum weekly income of £75 for single pensioners, will help drive up standards of health. So will our plans for annual winter fuel payments, the £150 million investment in home energy efficiency, and the availability this winter – for the first time – for flu jabs for all over 75-year-olds.

'Low wages are a health hazard. So we are improving health by introducing a National Minimum Wage, putting money into the pockets and handbags of the worst off who are in work.

'Bad housing makes people ill. So we are investing £5 billion over the lifetime of this Parliament in improving existing homes and building better new homes.

'Being out of work is bad for your health. Our New Deal financed from the Windfall Levy has helped over 400,000 extra people into jobs.

'By next April, 13 million people will be helped in 26 Health Action Zones, designed specifically to tackle health inequalities in areas including inner cities, coalfield communities, struggling rural areas, and places where wealth and poverty live cheek by jowl.

'More than £3 billion under the New Deal for Regeneration will help regener-
ate the most deprived areas. Within this, £800 million will be made available
under the New Deal for Communities to help some of the country's most
deprived neighbourhoods.

'The Integrated Transport White Paper will help ensure that public transport will be a weapon to help alleviate poverty, improve access to jobs and
strengthen communities. The Social Exclusion Unit will continue to co-ordinate
a national drive to support people who have been cut off from the mainstream
of society.

'As the report points out, tackling health inequalities will require action
across the whole of Government, but there is an important role for the Department of Health. Modernising the health service and ensuring fair access to
services is a vital component of that effort – backed up with a £21 billion boost
over the next three years. Health Action Zones are already at work on tackling
health inequalities in their areas and there will be a network of healthy living
centres across the country, working on the ground to improve the health of
the worst off in society. We will also be publishing soon our White Paper on
tobacco with action focused on the socially disadvantaged who are most likely
to smoke.

'The Green Paper, *Our Healthier Nation*, made clear our commitment to tackling health inequalities. . . . Inequalities which have persisted throughout the
century and often worsened in the past two decades will not be swept away
overnight. Sir Donald's work will be a key influence on our long-term strategy
to narrow the health gap.'

REFERENCES

Acheson, D. (1998) *Report into Inequalities in Health*, London, Department of Health.

Adams, R. (1996) *The Personal Social Services*, London, Longman.

Adler, M., Petch, A. and Tweedie, J. (1989) *Parental Choice and Educational Policy*, Edinburgh, Edinburgh University Press.

Ahmed, Y. (1996) 'Health promotion, quasi-markets and the NHS', in Braddon, D. and Foster, D. (eds) *Privatisation: Social Science Themes and Perspectives*, Dartmouth Publishing Co., pp. 67–94.

Alcock, P. (1997) 'Consolidation or stagnation? Social policy under the Major governments', in May, M., Brunsdon, E. and Craig, G. (eds) *Social Policy Review* **9**, 17–33.

Allsop, J. (1995) *Health Policy and the NHS: Towards 2000*, London, Longman.

Allsop, J. (1997) 'Why health care should be provided free at the point of service', in Gladstone, D. (ed.) *How to Pay for Health Care*, London, Institute of Economic Affairs, pp. 7–15.

Ambler, J. (1997) 'Who benefits from educational choice? Some evidence from Europe', in Cohn, E. (ed.) *Market Approaches to Education: Vouchers and School Choice*, Oxford, Pergamon, pp. 353–80.

Atkinson, A.B. and Micklewright, J. (1989) 'Turning the screw: benefits for the unemployed, 1979–88', in Atkinson, A.B. (ed.) *Poverty and Social Security*, Hemel Hempstead, Harvester Wheatsheaf, pp. 125–57.

Audit Commission (1996) *Balancing the Care Equation*, London, HMSO.

Baggott, R. (1994) *Health and Health Care in Britain*, London, Macmillan.

Bagley, C. (eds) (1997) *Choice and Diversity in Schooling: Perspectives and Prospects*, London, Routledge, pp. 7–28.

Baker, W. (1997) 'DTI Review', Report to Anti-Poverty Sub Committee of Liverpool City Council, Liverpool.

Balchin, P. and Rhoden, M. (1998) *Housing: The Essential Foundations*, London, Routledge.

Balchin, P., Issac, D. and Rhoden, M. (1998) 'Housing policy and finance', in Balchin, P. and Rhoden, M. (1998) *Housing: The Essential Foundations*, London, Routledge, pp. 50–106.

Baldock, J. and Ungerson, C. (1994) *Becoming Consumers of Community Care*, York, Joseph Rowntree Foundation.

Baldwin, S. (1997) 'Charging for community care', *Social Policy Review* **9**.

Baldwin, S. and Lunt, N. (1996) *Local Authority Charging Policies for Community Care*, Social Care Research 88, York, Joseph Rowntree Foundation.

Ball, S. (1990) *Education, Inequality and School Reform: Values in Crisis! An Inaugural Lecture*, London, King's College.

Barnett, C. (1986) *The Audit of War*, London, Macmillan.

Barr, N., Glennerster, H. and Le Grand, J. (1989) *Working for Patients? The Right Approach*, Welfare State Programme, London, London School of Economics.

Barrow, M. (1998) 'Financing of schools: a national or local quasi-market?', in Bartlett, W., Roberts, J.A. and Le Grand, J. (1998) *A Revolution in Social Policy: Quasi-market Reforms in the 1990s*, Bristol, Policy Press, pp. 63–77.

Bartlett, W., Roberts, J.A. and Le Grand, J. (1998) *A Revolution in Social Policy: Quasi-market Reforms in the 1990s*, Bristol, Polity Press.

Becker, S. (1997) *Responding to Poverty: The Politics of Cash and Care*, London, Longman.

Benefit Agency (1995) *What to Do after a Death in England and Wales*, Benefit Agency, London.

Bevan, A. (1978 [first published 1952]) *In Place of Fear*, London, Quartet.

Beveridge, W. (1942) *Social Insurance and Allied Services Report*, Cmd. 6404, HMSO, London.

Beveridge, W. (1948) *Voluntary Action: A Report of Methods of Social Advance*, London, Allen & Unwin.

Birch, S. (1986) 'Increasing patient charges in the National Health Service: a method of privatizing primary care', *Journal of Social Policy* **15**(2), 163–8.

Birmingham Settlement, Community Energy Research and the Bristol Energy Centre (1993) *The Hidden Disconnected: An Investigation of Consumer, Fuel Company and Agency Responses to Prepayment Meters and Fuel Direct*, Birmingham.

Bishop, M. and Kay, J. (1988) *Does Privatisation Work? Lessons from the UK*, London, London Business School.

Borrie, G. (1994) *Social Justice: Strategies for National Renewal*, Report of the Commission on Social Justice, London, Vintage.

Bowe, R., Ball, S.J. and Gold, A. (1993) *Reforming Education and Changing Schools*, London, Routledge.

Bradshaw, J. (1992) 'Social Security', in Marsh, D. and Rhodes, R.A.W. (eds) *Implementing Thatcherite Policies: Audit of an Era*, Buckingham, Open University Press, pp. 81–99.

Brown, J. (1995) *The British Welfare State: A Critical History*, Oxford, Blackwell.

Burchardt, T. (1997) *Boundaries between Public and Private Welfare: A Typology and Map of Services*, CASEpaper 2, London, Centre for Analysis of Social Exclusion, London School of Economics.

Burchardt, T. and Hills, J. (1997) *Private Welfare Insurance and Social Security: Pushing the Boundaries*, York, York Publishing Services Ltd.

Butcher, T. (1995) *Delivering Welfare; the Governance of the Social Services in the 1990s*, Buckingham, Open University Press.

Butler, E., Pirie, M. and Young, P. (1985) *The Omega File*, London, Adam Smith Institute.

Butler, J. (1993) 'A case study in the National Health Service: working for patients,' in Taylor-Gooby, P. and Lawson, R. (eds) (1993) *Markets and Managers*, Buckingham, Open University Press, pp. 54–68.

Butler, S. (1998) *Access Denied: The Exclusion of People in Need from Social Housing*, London, Shelter.

Callaghan, J. (1992) 'The Educational Debate', in Williams, M., Daugherty R. and Banks F. (eds) *Continuing the Education Debate*, London, Cassell, pp. 9–16.

Calvert, H. (1978) *Social Security Law*, London, Sweet & Maxwell.

Centre for Public Services (1997) *Reinventing Government in Britain: The Performance of Next Steps Agencies. Implications for the USA.* Sheffield.

Charlesworth, J., Clarke, J. and Cochrane, A. (1996) 'Tangled webs? Managing local mixed economies of care', *Public Administration*, **74**, 67–88.

Chubb, J. and Moe, T. (1990) *Politics, Markets and America's Schools*, Washington DC, Brookings Institute.

Clapham, D., Munro, M. and Kay, H. (1994) *Financing User Choice in Housing and Community Care*, Housing Summary 6, York, Joseph Rowntree Foundation.

Cohen, R. and Tarpey, M. (eds) (1988) *Single Payments – the Disappearing Safety Net*, Poverty Pamphlet No. 74, London, CPAG.

Cohen, R., Ferres, G., Hollins, C., Long, G. and Smith R. (1996) *Out of Pocket: Failure of the Social Fund*, London, Children's Society.

Cole, I. and Furbey, R. (1994) *The Eclipse of Council Housing*, London, Routledge.

Common, R. and Flynn, N. (1992) *Contracting For Care*, York, Joseph Rowntree Foundation.

Cooper, M. and Culyer, A.J. (1971) 'An economic survey of the nature and intent of the British National Health Service', *Social Science and Medicine*, **5**(1), 1–13.

Cox, C. (1988) 'What makes people like us tick?', *Times Educational Supplement*, 16 September.

Craig, G. (1992) 'Managing the poorest: the Social Fund in context', in Carter, P., Jeffs, T. and Smith, M.K. (eds) *Changing Social Work and Welfare*, Buckingham, Open University Press, pp. 65–80.

Craig, G. (1993) 'Classification and control: the role of Social Fund loans', in Howells, G., Crow, I. and Moroney, M. (eds) *Aspects of Credit and Debt*, London, Sweet & Maxwell, pp. 109–30.

Craig, G. (1998) 'The privatisation of human misery', *Critical Social Policy* **18**(1), 51–76.

Craig, G. and Dowler, E. (1997) 'Let them eat cake! Poverty, hunger and the UK state', in Riches, G. (ed.) *First World Hunger: Food Security and Welfare*, Basingstoke, Macmillan, pp. 108–133.

Dale, R. (1989) 'The Thatcherite Project in Education: the case of the City Technology Colleges', *Critical Social Policy* **9**(3), 4–19.

Dale, R. (1997) 'Educational markets and school choice', *British Journal of Sociology of Education*, **18**(3), 451–68.

David, N., West, A. and Ribbens, J. (1994) *Mother's Intuition? Choosing Secondary Schools*, London, Falmer Press.

Davies, B. (1997) 'Equity and efficiency in community care: from muddle to model and model to . . . ?', *Policy and Politics*, **25**(4), 337–59.

Deacon, A. (1997) '"Welfare to work": options and issues', in May, M., Brunsdon, E. and Craig, G. (eds) *Social Policy Review* **9**, London, Social Policy Association.

Deakin, N. (1996) 'The devils in the detail: some reflections on contracting for social care by voluntary organisations', *Social Policy and Administration*, **30**(1), 20–38.

Deakin, N. and Walsh, K. (1996) 'The enabling state: the role of markets and contracts', *Public Administration*, **74**, 33–48.

Deakin, N. and Parry, R. (1998) 'The treasury and New Labour's social policy', in *Social Policy Review* **10**, Social Policy Association, London, pp. 34–56.

Dean, H. (1993) 'Social security: the income maintenance business', in Taylor-Gooby, P. and Lawson, R. (eds) *Markets and Managers*, Buckingham, Open University Press, pp. 85–101.

Department of Education and Science (1986) *City Technology Colleges: A New Choice of School*, London, DES.

Department of Education and Science (1987) *Admission of Pupils to Maintained Schools: A Consultation Paper*, London, HMSO.

Department of Education and Science (1992) *The Government's Expenditure Plans 1991/2 to 1993/4*, Cmd. 1511, London, HMSO.

Department for Education (DfE/Welsh Office) (1992) *Choice and Diversity: A New Framework for Schools*, London, HMSO.

Department for Education and Employment (1997) Press Release, 15 October.

Department for Education and Employment (1997a) 'No government department's work is more important, David Blunkett', 100/97, 14 May.

Department for Education and Employment (1997b) 'New plans for nursery education as vouchers are scrapped – Estelle Morris', 197/97, 14 July.

Department for Education and Employment (1997c) 'Blunkett announces £200 million homework clubs plans', 418/97, 8 December.

Department for Education and Employment (1997d) 'Blackstone outlines proposals for home-school contracts', 250/97, 11 August.

Department for Education and Employment (1997e) 'Estelle Morris calls for sharper focus on basics in primary schools', 135/97, 10 June.

Department for Education and Employment (1997f) 'Blunkett sets tough new national targets to boost three Rs', 96/97, 13 May.

Department for Education and Employment (1997g) 'Tough new tests will raise standards – Blackstone', 252/97, 11 August.

Department for Education and Employment (1997h) 'Class size reductions to enhance parental choice and support quality education – Byers', 209/98, 27 April.

Department for Education and Employment (1997i) 'Estelle Morris pledges more school performance information', 156/97, 25 June.

Department for Education and Employment (1997j) 'Diversity and specialism will boost standards – Blunkett', 351/97, 5 November.

Department for Education and Employment (1997k) 'Blunkett outlines tough new measures on failing schools', 280/97, 2 June.

Department for Education and Employment (1997l) 'Crackdown on failing teachers – Byers', 118/97, 28 May.

Department for Education and Employment (1997m) 'Byers calls for fast-track sacking of worst teachers', 215/97, 18 July.

Department for Education and Employment (1997n) 'Super teachers are key to our standards crusade – Blunkett', 246/97, 6 August.

Department for Education and Employment (1997o) 'Local education authorities must raise standards – Blunkett', 144/97, 12 June.

Department for Education and Employment (1997p) 'Byers announces first decisions on grant-maintained status', 109/97, 20 May.

Department for Education and Employment (1997q) 'Burying old prejudices with £500,000 boost for private/state school partnerships – Byers', 393/97, 26 November.

Department for Education and Employment (1997r) 'Action zones head radical bill for raising standards – Blunkett', 412/97, 4 December.

Department for Education and Employment (1997s) 'Public private partnerships key to tackling crumbling schools – Blunkett', 152/97, 23 June.

Department for Education and Employment (1997t) 'Blunkett welcomes 2 billion pound new deal for schools', 2/97, 2 July.

Department for Education and Employment (1997u) 'Minister sees plans for country's first private finance initiative school', 89/97, 9 July.

Department for Education and Employment (1998) 'Admission appeals for maintained primary and secondary schools by local education authority area in England', 443/98, 25 September.

Department for Education and Employment (1998a) 'Howells Announces Result of Student Loan Debt Sale', 115/98, 5 March.

Department for Education and Employment (1998b) 'Early Years Places on Target for Four Year Olds', 154/98, 27 March.

Department for Education and Employment (1998c) 'Byers details first 51 numeracy summer schools', 293/98, 9 June.

Department for Education and Employment (1998d) 'Permanent exclusions from schools in England 1996/97 and exclusion appeals lodged by parents in England 1996/97', 451/98, 30 September.

Department for Education and Employment (1998e) '£500m will help schools and LEAs to reduce truancy and exclusions – Estelle Morris', 483/98, 22 October.

Department for Education and Employment (1998f) 'Byers announces action to stop schools using exclusions to enhance performance table scores', 361/98, 13 July.

Department for Education and Employment (1998g) 'Blunkett launches homework clubs and guidance', 194/98, 21 April.

Department for Education and Employment (1998h) 'Partnerships with parents show the way forward – Blunkett', 16/98, 15 March.

Department for Education and Employment (1998i) 'Byers outlines plans for new 100 per cent delegation', 271/98, 29 May.

Department for Education and Employment (1998j) 'Action on surplus places to boost standards and parental choice – Byres', 103/98, 26 February.

Department for Education and Employment (1998k) 'Early assessment will help give children best possible start at school – Clarke', 412/98, 3 September.

Department for Education and Employment (1998l) 'Five-yearly inspection cycle for education authorities – Byres', 30/98, 22 January.

Department for Education and Employment (1998m) 'Councils get tough new English test targets – Byers', 5/98, 7 January.

Department for Education and Employment (1998n) '£1 million to foster links with independent schools – Morris', 459/98, 7 October.

Department for Education and Employment (1998o) 'Fourth major education act this century – Balfour, Butler, Baker and Now Blunkett', 382/98, 27 July.

Department for Education and Employment (1998p) 'Multi-million boost for education action zones – Blunkett', 199/98, 23 April.

Department for Education and Employment (1998q) '£19 billion boost for education', 360/98, 14 July.

Department for Education and Employment (1998r) 'Morris announces expansion to 500 specialist schools', 496/98, 29 October.

Department for Education and Employment (1998s) 'Byers reveals first beacon schools in £1.8 million plan to share education expertise', 351/98, 7 July.

Department for Education and Employment (1998t) 'Establishment of up to 100 beacon schools to raise standards – Byers', 215/98, 30 April.

Department for Education and Employment (1998u) '£11 million sponsorship boost for specialist schools', 100/98, 25 February.

Department for Education and Employment (1998v) 'Biggest ever specialist school expansion – Morris', 304/98, 16 June.

Department for Education and Employment (1998w) 'PPP deals worth £27 million signed – Howells', 91/98, 18 February.

Department for Education and Employment (1999a) 'Blunkett unveils £60 million bonus scheme for schools', 20/99, 19 January.

Department for Education and Employment (1999b) 'Blunkett issues tough challenge to education authorities', 9/99, 8 January.

Department of Health (1988) *Health and Personal Social Services Statistics for England*, 1988 edn, London, HMSO.

Department of Health (1989) *Working for Patients*, London, HMSO.

Department of Health (1994) *Hospital Activity Statistics: England 1983–1994*, Statistical Bulletin, London, Department of Health.

Department of Health (1997a) 'Minister warns council: government ready to intervene', 97/277, 15 October.

Department of Health (1997b) 'Action taken to achieve right balance for adoption', 98/353, 28 August.

Department of Health (1997c) 'Plans for psychiatric hospital closures to be vetted by new group', 97/222, 12 September.

Department of Health (1997d) 'New guidance promised on help for families of psychiatric patients', 97/396, 12 December.

Department of Health (1997e) 'NHS savings targeted by new task force', 97/132, 11 June.

Department of Health (1997f) Alan Milburn publishes private finance data and pledges greater openness', 97/126, 9 June.

Department of Health (1997g) 'Board meetings of NHS trusts to be opened to the public', 97/148, 30 June.

Department of Health (1997h) 'NHS secrecy to be swept aside – Alan Milburn', 97/371, 2 December.

Department of Health (1997i) '8th wave fundholding deferred', 97/103, 20 May.

Department of Health (1997j) 'Fairness and equity for hospital treatment', 97/169, 16 July.

Department of Health (1997k) 'Alan Milburn launches programme of GP commissioning pilots', 97/146, 26 June.

Department of Health (1997l) 'New partnerships for improved health services', 97/253, 30 September.

Department of Health (1997m) ' "Health action zones" envisaged as cooperative NHS partnerships', 97/145, 25 June.

Department of Health (1997n) 'Frank Dobson announces action to "end the two tier National Health Service" ', 97/091, 9 May.

Department of Health (1997o) 'New mission to tackle inequalities that lead to ill-health – Tessa Jowell', 97/095, 15 May.

Department of Health (1997p) 'Tessa Jowell pledges action to tackle health divide', 97/214, 8 September.

Department of Health (1997q) 'Cash formula to help tackle health inequalities', 97/220, 11 September.

Department of Health (1997r) 'High quality, not "bean counting" to be central NHS priority – Baroness Jay', 97/234, 19 September.

Department of Health (1997s) 'NHS needs, not market whim, to drive hospital building plans: Milburn', 97/380, 5 December.

Department of Health (1997t) '£300 million cash boost for NHS', 97/274, 14 October.

Department of Health (1997u) '£300 million lottery cash to fund healthy living centres', 97/409, 18 December.

Department of Health (1997v) '£80 million out of red tape and into the front line', 97/414, 22 December.

Department of Health (1997w) 'Doctors and nurses should be in the NHS driving seat', 97/372, 3 December.

Department of Health (1997x) 'NHS pensions mis-selling still unresolved', 97/197, 19 August.

Department of Health (1997y) 'New deposit scheme to redress NHS pensions mis-selling', 97/321, 3 November.

Department of Health (1998a) 'Statistics published on social services spending', 98/241, 18 June.

Department of Health (1998b) 'Key statistics of social services', 98/408, 30 September.

Department of Health (1998c) 'Statistics on children's homes at 31 March 1997, England', 98/039, 29 January.

Department of Health (1998d) 'Children looked after by local authorities 1997', 98/302, 23 July.

218

Department of Health (1998e) 'Figures published on children looked after by councils', 98/421, 8 October.

Department of Health (1998f) 'Report calls on council to act immediately to protect children', 98/232, 11 June.

Department of Health (1998g) 'Social services failing children in care, says Inspectorate', 98/387, 21 September.

Department of Health (1998h) 'Children's homes: improving quality of care', 98/0527, 18 November.

Department of Health (1998i) 'New plans to bridge gulf between health and social care', 98/381, 16 September.

Department of Health (1998j) 'Health secretary pledges to transform children's services', 98/388, 21 September.

Department of Health (1998k) 'Nursing homes and private health care to face open regulation', 98/019, 19 January.

Department of Health (1998l) 'They look after their own, don't they?', 98/061, 18 February.

Department of Health (1998m) 'Statistics on in-patients detained under the Mental Health Act', 98/0553 November.

Department of Health (1998n) *Modernising Health and Social Services*, White Paper, London, Department of Health.

Department of Health (1998o) 'Joint guidance for the NHS and social services for the first time ever', 98/404, 30 September.

Department of Health (1998p) *Partnership in Action: New Opportunities for Joint Working between Health and Social Services*, London, Department of Health.

Department of Health (1998q) 'Figures published on patients detained under Mental Health Act', 98/041, 29 January.

Department of Health (1998r) 'Expert advisor appointed to start review of Mental Health Act', 98/391, 22 September.

Department of Health (1998s) Frank Dobson outlines Third Way for mental health', 98/311, 29 July.

Department of Health (1998t) *Modernising Mental Health Services*, London, Department of Health.

Department of Health (1998u) 'Health secretary outlines reform of social services system', 98/0557, 30 November.

Department of Health (1998v) 'NHS to save up to £45 million on commercial insurance premiums', 98/345, 20 August.

Department of Health (1998w) 'NHS still the envy of the world', 98/0447, 22 October.

Department of Health (1998x) 'NHS charges', 98/078, 2 March.

Department of Health (1998y) 'Health action zone bids focus on improving elderly, children's and mental health services', 98/054, 9 February.

Department of Health (1998z) 'Fifteen new health action zones to tackle health inequalities', 98/329, 11 August.

Department of Health (1998aa) 'One million children from deprived areas set to gain from extra £10 million NHS dentistry package', 98/114, 27 March.

Department of Health (1998bb) 'All health authorities get cash boost in £31 billion funding allocations', 98/0500, 10 November.

Department of Health and Social Security (1980) *Public Expenditure White Paper*, London, HMSO.

Department of Health and Social Security (1985) *Reform of Social Security*, Green Paper, Cmd. 9517, London, DHSS.

Department of the Environment (1987) *Housing: The Government's Proposals*, Cmd. 214, London, HMSO.

Department of the Environment (1996) *Housing and Construction Statistics 1979–82*, London, HMSO.

Department of the Environment, Transport and the Regions (1997a) 'Housing is no longer the missing piece of the jigsaw – Hilary Armstrong', 244/ENV, 27 June.

Department of the Environment, Transport and the Regions (1997b) 'Local government – agent for development and social justice', 294/ENV, 23 July.

Department of the Environment, Transport and the Regions (1997c) 'Housing Plus: Towards the Millenium and Beyond', 358/ENV, 17 September.

Department of the Environment, Transport and the Regions (1997d) 'Government vote of confidence for investors in private rented housing and responsible landlords', 237/ENV, 24 June.

Department of the Environment, Transport and the Regions (1997e) 'Chancellor releases new resources for housing', DETR 2, 2 July.

Department of the Environment, Transport and the Regions (1997f) 'Hilary Armstrong urges councils to keep rent increases down', 464/ENV, 26 November.

Department of the Environment, Transport and the Regions (1997g) 'Councils' public private partnerships get triple boost', 462/ENV 19 November.

Department of the Environment, Transport and the Regions (1997h) 'New powers to combat antisocial behaviour', 335/ENV, 1 September.

Department of the Environment, Transport and the Regions (1997i) 'Tackling homelessness: it cannot be done in isolation', 505/ENV, 10 December.

Department of the Environment, Transport and the Regions (1998a) 'Hilary Armstrong defines role of government in the modern housing market', 488/ENV, 16 June.

Department of the Environment, Transport and the Regions (1998b) 'Investing in housing and regeneration for the next millennium', 611/ENV, 22 July.

Department of the Environment, Transport and the Regions (1998c) 'More Local Government PFI projects get green light', 519/ENV, 24 June.

Department of the Environment, Transport and the Regions (1998d) 'Tenants to benefit in government transfer programme', 207/ENV, 19 March.

Department of the Environment, Transport and the Regions (1998e) '£248 million government funding to help build thriving communities'. 113/ENV, 19 February.

Department of the Environment, Transport and the Regions (1998f) 'Delivering Quality Local Services', 872/ENV, 24 September.

Department of Social Security (1994) *Personal Pension Statistics 1992/3*, Revised edition, London, Government Statistical Service.

Department of Social Security (1997a) 'Harman takes first step towards tackling poverty and division', 97/074, 28 May.

Department of Social Security (1997b) 'Harman highlights work as the best form of welfare', 97/059, 6 May.

Department of Social Security (1997c) 'Harriet Harman sets out her goals for steering social security towards the millennium', 97/077, 2 June.

Department of Social Security (1997d) 'New ideas seminar marks "turning point" on fraud', 97/184, 23 September.

Department of Social Security (1997e) 'Swift and substantial progress in pensions review', 97/186, 24 September.

Department of Social Security (1998a) 'Contracts awarded for benefits agency medical service', 98/033, 19 February.

Department of Social Security (1998b) 'Benefit fraud inspectorate is welfare reform in action, says Harman', 98/215, 22 July.

Department of Social Security (1998c) 'Recovery of money fraudulently claimed in benefits', 98/141, 2 June.

Department of Social Security (1998d) *A New Contract for Welfare: Partnership in Pension*, Green Paper, London, Department of Social Security.

Department of Social Security (1998e) 'Poorest pensioners big winners in £2.5 billion pensions boost, says Harman', 98/209, 17 July.

Department of Social Security (1999a) 'New priorities for welfare reform', 99/001, 6 January.

Department of Social Security (1999b) 'Blunkett and Darling welcome £80 million cash boost for new welfare reform programme', 13/99, 13 January.

Donnison, D. (1984) 'The progressive potential of privatisation', in Le Grand, J. and Robinson, R. (eds) *Privatisation and the Welfare State*, London, Allen & Unwin.

Doran, N. (1994) 'Risky business: codifying embodied experience in the Manchester unity of oddfellows', *Journal of Historial Sociology*, **7**(4), 131–154.

Drakeford, M. (1993) 'But who will do the work?', *Critical Social Policy*, **38**(2), 64–76.

Drakeford, M. (1995) *Token Gesture: A Report on the Use of Token Meters by the Gas, Electricity and Water Companies*, Wales Office, Pontypool, National Local Government Forum Against Poverty.

Drakeford, M. (1997a) 'The poverty of privatisation', *Critical Social Policy*, **51**, 115–32.

Drakeford, M. (1997b) *Funeral, Poverty and the Social Fund*, Barry, Wales Local Government Anti-Poverty Forum.

DSS (1995) *Social Security Departmental Report, The Government's Expenditure Plans 1995–96 to 1997–98*, London, HMSO.

Edwards, T. and Whitty, G. (1997) 'Marketing quality: traditional and modern versions of educational excellence', in Glatter, R., Woods, P.A. and Bagley, C. (eds) *Choice and Diversity in Schooling: Perspectives and Prospects*, London, Routledge, pp. 29–43.

Edwards, T., Gewirtz, S. and Whitty, G. (1994) 'Whose choice of schools? Making sense of City Technology Colleges', in Arnot, M. and Barton, L. (eds) *Voicing Concerns: Sociological Perspectives on Contemporary Education Reforms*, London, Triangle, pp. 143–62.

Enthoven, A. (1985) *Reflections on the Management of the National Health Service*, London, Nuffield Provincial Hospitals Trust.

Ernst, J. (1994) *Whose Utility? The Social Impact of Public Utility Privatization and Regulation in Britain*, Milton Keynes, Open University Press.

Evans, M. (1997) 'Means testing flaws', *New Economy*, **4**(2), 89–94.

Evans, J. and Vincent, C. (1997) 'Parental choice and special education', in Glatter, R., Woods, P.A. and Bagley, C. (eds) *Choice and Diversity in Schooling: Perspectives and Prospects*, London, Routledge, pp. 102–15.

Evers, A. (1993) 'The welfare mix approach: understanding the pluralism of welfare systems', in Evers, A. and Svetlik, I. (eds) *Balancing Pluralism; New Welfare Mixes in Care for the Elderly*, Aldershot, Averbury.

Fawcett, H. (1995) 'The privatisation of welfare: the impact of parties on the private/public mix in pension provision', *West European Politics*, **18**(4), 150–69.

Field, F. (1998) 'The Beveridge Memorial Lecture', http://www.dss.gov.uk/hq/press/speeches/ff18298.htm

Finer Jones, C. (1997) 'The new social policy in Britain', *Social Policy and Administration*, **31**(5), 154–70.

Fitz, J., Power, S. and Halpin, D. (1993) 'Opting for grant maintained status: a study of policymaking in education' *Policy Studies*, **14**(1), 4–20.

Fitzpatrick, T. (1998) 'The rise of market collectivism', in Brunsdon, E., Dean, H. and Woods, R. (eds) *Social Policy Review 10*, London, Social Policy Association, pp. 13–33.

Flude, M. and Hammer, M. (1990) 'Opting for an uncertain future', in Flude, M. and Hammer, M. (eds) *The Education Reform Act, 1988: Its Origins and Implications*, Basingstoke, Falmer Press, pp. 51–72.

Ford, J. (1997) 'Mortgage arrears, mortgage possessions and homelessness', in Burrows, R., Pleace, N. and Quilgars, D. (eds) *Homelessness and Social Policy*, London, Routledge, pp. 88–108.

Ford, J. and Kempson, E. (1997) *Bridging the Gap? Safety Net for Mortgage Borrowers*, York, Joseph Rowntree Foundation.

Forrest, R. (1993) 'Contracting housing provision: competition and privatisation in the housing sector', in Taylor-Gooby, P. and Lawson, R. (eds) *Markets and Managers*, Buckingham, Open University Press, pp. 38–53.

Forrest, R. and Murie, A. (1993) *Selling the Welfare State: The Privatisation of Public Housing*, London, Routledge.

Foster, C. (1994) 'Rival explanations of public ownership, its failure and privatisation', *Public Administration*, **72**, 489–503.

Fraser, T. (1984) *The Evolution of the British Welfare State*, London, Macmillan.

Garnham, A. and Knights, E. (1994) *Putting the Treasury First: 'The Truth about Child Support'*, London, Child Poverty Action Group.

Gas Consumer Council (1997) *Report on the GCC Prepayment Seminar*, 28 April, London, GCC.

Gewirtz, S., Ball, S.J. and Bowe, R. (1995) *Markets, Choice and Equity in Education*, Buckingham, Open University Press.

Giddens, A. (1998) 'The future of the welfare state', in Novak, M. (ed.) *Is There a Third Way: Essays on the Changing Direction of Socialist Thought*, London, Institute of Economic Affairs, pp. 25–9.

Gladstone, D. (ed.) (1997) *How to Pay for Health Care*, London, Institute of Economic Affairs.

Glatter, R., Woods, P.A. and Bagley, C. (1997a) 'Diversity, differentiation and hierarchy: school choice and parental preference', in Glatter, R., Woods, P.A. and Bagley, C. (eds) *Choice and Diversity in Schooling: Perspectives and Prospects*, London, Routledge, pp. 7–28.

Glatter, R., Woods, P.A. and Bagley, C. (1997b) 'Review and implications', in Glatter, R., Woods, P.A. and Bagley, C. (eds) *Choice and Diversity in Schooling: Perspectives and Prospects*, London, Routledge, pp. 191–205.

Glennerster, H. (1992) *Paying for Welfare: Issues for the Nineties*, Welfare State Programme Paper No. 82, London, London School of Economics.

Glennerster, H. (1996) 'Vouchers and quasi vouchers in education', in May, M., Brunsdon, E. and Craig, G. (eds) *Social Policy Review* **8**, London, Social Policy Association, pp. 125–37.

Glennerster, H. and Hills, J. (eds) (1998) *The State of Welfare: The Economics of Social Spending*, Oxford, Oxford University Press.

Goldsmith, M. (1997) 'Co-payment: a vehicle for NHS funding enhancement', in Gladstone, D. (ed.) *How to Pay for Health Care*, London, Institute of Economic Affairs, pp. 16–22.

Goodwin, J. (1998) 'Locked out', *Roof*, July/August, 25–9.

Graham, S. (1997) 'Liberalised utilities, new technologies and urban social polarization: the UK experience', *European Urban and Regional Studies*, **4**(2), 135–50.

Grantovetter, M. and Swedberg, R. (1992) *The Sociology of Economic Life*, Oxford, Westview Press.

Gray, J. (1996) *School Effectiveness and School Improvement*, Buckingham, Open University Press.

Green, D. (1996) 'Medical Case Without the State', in Seldon, A. (ed.) *Re-Privatising Welfare: After the Lost Century*. London, Institute of Economic Affairs.

Greer, P. (1994) *Transforming Central Government: the Next Steps Initiative*, Buckingham, Open University Press.

Griffiths, R. (1983) *NHS Management Inquiry*, London, Department of Health and Social Security.

Guy, S., Graham, S. and Marvin, S. (1997) 'Splintering networks: cities and technical networks in 1990s Britain', *Urban Studies*, **34**(2), 191–216.

Haines, K. and Drakeford, M. (1998) *Young People and Youth Justice*, London, Macmillan.

Hall, S. (1998) 'The great moving nowhere show', *Marxism Today*, November/December, 9–14.

Halpin, D., Power, S. and Fitz, J. (1997) 'Opting into the past? Grant-maintained schools and the reinvention of tradition', in Glatter, R., Woods, P.A. and Bagley, C. (eds) *Choice and Diversity in Schooling: Perspectives and Prospects*, London, Routledge, pp. 59–70.

Ham, C.J. (1994) 'Reforming health services: learning from the UK experience', *Social Policy and Administration*, **28**(4).

Hansard, 12 June 1997: 'Social Security (Social Fund and Claims and Payments) (Miscellaneous Amendments) Regulations 1997', cols 1032–41.

Harding, T., Meredith, B. and Wistow, G. (eds) (1996) *Options for Long Term Care: Economic, Social and Ethical Choices*, London, HMSO.

Hargreaves, A. and Reynolds, D. (1989) 'Decomprehensivization', in Reynolds, D. and Hargreaves, A. (eds) *Education Policy: Controversy and Critiques*, Lewes, Falmer Press.

Harman, H. (1998) 'A modern anti-poverty strategy', speech at the Centenary Conference of Seebohm Rowntree's First Study of Poverty in York, DSS98/073.

Harriott, S. and Matthews, L. (1998) *Social Housing – An Introduction*, London, Longman.

Harris, J. (1977) *William Beveridge: A Biography*, Oxford, Clarendon Press.

Harris, M. (1986) *Looking at Voluntary Agencies*, RIPA Report, **7**(1), 11–12.

Harrison, S. (1988) *Managing the National Health Service: Shifting the Frontier?*, London, Chapman & Hall.

Hartley, K. (1990) 'Contracting-out in Britain: achievements and problems', in Richardson, J.J. (ed.) *Privatization and Deregulation in Canada and Britain*, Dartmouth, IRPP, pp. 177–98.

Hayden, C. (1997) *Children Excluded from Primary School: Debates, Evidence, Responses*, Buckingham, Open University Press.

Hayek, F. (1960) *The Constitution of Liberty*, London, Routledge & Kegan Paul.

Heald, D. (1989) 'The United Kingdom: privatisation and its political context', in Vickers, J. and Wright, V. (eds) *The Politics of Privatisation in Western Europe*, London, Cass, pp. 31–48.

Health Service Commissioner (1998) *Fifth Report for Session 1997–98*, London, HMSO.

Hendry, R. (1998) *Fair Shares for All? The Development of Needs Based Government Funding in Education, Health and Housing*, London, London School of Economics.

Henwood, M., Wistow, G. and Robinson, J. (1996) 'Halfway there? Policy, politics and outcomes in community care', *Social Policy and Administration*, **30**(1), 39–53.

Herbert, A. and Kempson, E. (1995) *Water Debt and Disconnection*, London, Policy Studies Institute.

Hill, M. (1990) *Social Security Policy in Britain*, Aldershot, Edward Elgar..

Hills, J. (1991) *Unravelling Housing Finance: Subsidies, Benefits and Taxation*, Oxford, Clarendon Press.

Hills, J. (1997) *The Future of Welfare: A Guide to the Debate*, York, Joseph Rowntree Foundation.

Hills, J. (1998) *Thatcherism, New Labour and the Welfare State*, London School of Economics, CASE paper 13.

Hirsch, F. (1977) *The Social Limits to Growth*, London, Routledge & Kegan Paul.

Hirschman, A.O. (1982) *Shifting Involvements: Private Interest and Public Action*, Oxford, Martin Robertson.

Hoggett, P. (1991) 'A new management for the public sector?', *Policy and Politics*, **19**, 243–56.

Hoggett, P. (1996) 'New modes of control in the public service', *Public Administration*, **74**, 9–32.

Houghton, T., Anderson, M., Baines, R. and Heijne, C. (1998) *Counting the Hidden Disconnected: A Research Study Conducted by the Centre for Sustainable Energy, National Right to Fuel Campaign*, Bristol, Unison.

House of Commons Health Committee (1995) *Long-Term Care: NHS Responsibilities for Meeting Continuing Health Care Needs*, First Report Session 1995–96, HC19-1.

Hoyes, L., Lart, R., Means, R. and Taylor, M. (1994) *Community Care in Transition*, York, Joseph Rowntree Foundation.

Huby, M. and Dix, G. (1992) *Evaluating the Social Fund*, DSS Research Report No. 9, London, HMSO.

Huby, M. and Walker, R. (1991) 'Adapting to the Social Fund', *Social Policy and Administration*, **25**(4), 329–49.

Hunter, D.J. (1997) *Desperately Seeking Solutions: Rationing Health Care*, London, Longman.

Hyams-Parish, T. (1995) *Banished to the Exclusion Zone – A Guide to School Exclusions and the Law*, Children's Legal Centre, University of Essex.

Jack, I. (1991) 'Social services and the ageing population 1970–1990', *Social Policy and Administration*, **25**(4), 284–99.

Jackson, P.M. and Waddhams Price, C. (1994) *Privatisation and Regulation: A Review of the Issues*, London, Longman.

Jacques, M. (1998) 'Leader', *Marxism Today*, November/December, 2–3.

Jenkins, K., Caines, K. and Jackson, A. (1988) *Improving Management in Government: The Next Steps – A report to the Prime Minister*, Efficiency Unit, London, HMSO.

Jonathan, R. (1989) 'Choice and control in education: parental rights and social justice', *British Journal of Educational Studies*, **37**(4).

Joseph, K. (1976) *Stranded on the Middle Ground? Reflections on Circumstances and Policies*, London, Centre for Policy Studies.

Joseph, K. and Sumption, J. (1979) *Equality*, London, John Murray.

Joseph Rowntree Foundation (1996) *Meeting the Costs of Continuing Care*, York, Joseph Rowntree Foundation.

Jowell, R. (ed.) (1997) *British Social Attitudes: The 14th Report: The End of Conservative Values?*, Aldershot, Ashgate.

Judge, K. and Matthews, J. (1980) *Charging for Social Care: A Study of Consumer Charges and the Personal Social Services*, London, Allen & Unwin.

Kemp, P. (1992) 'Housing', in Marsh, D. and Rhodes, R.A.W. (eds) *Implementing Thatcherite Policies: Audit of an Era*, Buckingham, Open University Press, pp. 65–80.

Kempson, E. (1997) *Local Variations in Costs*, Social Policy Research, **123**, York, Joseph Rowntree Foundation.

Kendall, I., Blackmore, M., Bradshaw, Y., Jenkinson, S. and Johnson, N. (1997) 'Quality services in quasi-markets', in May, M., Brunsdon, E. and Craig, G. (eds) *Social Policy Review*, **9**, 184–202.

Kirkpatrick, I. and Lucio, M.M. (1996) 'Introduction: the contract state and the future of public management', *Public Administration*, **74**, 1–8.

Labour Party (1997) *Protecting Our Communities*. London, The Labour Party.

Labour Research (1997a) 'Tories fail pre-school test', *Labour Research*, **86**(1), 19–21.

Labour Research (1997b) 'Thank you Sid and goodbye!', *Labour Research*, March, 23–4.

Laing, W. (1998) *A Fair Price for Care? Disparities between Market Rates and State Funding of Residential Care*, York, Joseph Rowntree Foundation.

Laing and Buisson (1995) *Care of Elderly People: Market Survey 1995*, London, Laing and Buisson Publications.

Land, H. and Ward, S. (1985) *Women Won't Benefit: The Impact of the Social Security Bill on Women's Rights*, London, NCCL.

Langan, M. (1990) 'Community care in the 1990s: the community care White Paper: "Caring for People"', *Critical Social Policy*, **29**, 58–70.

Lapsley, I. and Llewellyn, S. (1998) 'Markets, hierarchies and choices in social care', in Bartlett, W., Roberts, J.A. and Le Grand, J. (eds) *A Revolution in Social Policy: Quasi-market Reforms in the 1990s*, Bristol, Policy Press, pp. 133–52.

Le Grand, J. (1993) 'Paying for or providing welfare?', in Page, R. and Deakin, N. (eds) *The Costs of Welfare*, Aldershot, Avebury, pp. 87–106.

Le Grand, J. (1997) 'Knights, knaves or pawns? Human behaviour and social policy', *Journal of Social Policy*, **26**(2), 149–70.

Lees, D. (1965) 'Health through choice', in Harris, R. (ed.) *Freedom or Free For All? Essays in Welfare, Trade and Choice*, London, Institute of Economic Affairs.

Legard, R., Ritchie, J. and Finch, H. (1998) *Older People and Income Support: Barriers and Triggers to the Take-up of Income Support*, London, Department of Social Security, Social Research Branch.

Letwin, O. (1988) *Privatising the World: A Study of International Privatisation in Theory and Practice*, London, Cassell Educational.

Levenson, R. (1992) 'Patients and the market in health care', *Critical Public Health*, **3**(1), 26–34.

Lewis, J. (with Bernstock, P., Bovwell, V. and Wookey, F.) (1996) 'The purchaser/provider split in social care: Is it working?, in *Social Policy and Administration*, **30**(1), 1–19.

Lilley, P. (1993) *Benefits and Costs: Securing the Future of Social Security*, Mais Lecture, City University Business School.

Lilley, P. (1995) *Winning the Welfare Debate*, London, Social Market Foundation.

Linneman, P.D. and Megbolugbe, I.F. (1994) 'Privatisation and housing policy', *Urban Studies*, **31**(4/5), 635–51.

Lister, R. (1996) 'Permanent revolution: the politics of two decades of social security reform', Paper presented to the DSS Summer School, King's College Cambridge.

Lloyd, J. (1998) 'Serfs no more', in Novak, M. (ed.) *Is There a Third Way: Essays on the Changing Direction of Socialist Thought*, London, Institute of Economic Affairs, pp. 30–6.

Local Government Anti-Poverty Unit (1995) *Survey of Charges for Social Care 1993–95*, London, Association of Metropolitan Authorities.

Loughlin, M. and Scott, C. (1997) 'The regulatory state', in Dunleavy, P., Gamble, A., Holliday, I. and Peele, G. (eds) *Developments in British Politics*, pp. 205–19.

Lowe, R. (1993) *The Welfare State in Britain Since 1945*, London, Macmillan.

Lund, B. (1996) *Housing Problems and Housing Policy*, London, Longman.

Lunt, N., Mannion, R. and Smith, P. (1996) 'Economic discourse and the market: the case of community care', *Public Administration*, **74**, 369–91.

Malpass, P. (1998) 'Housing policy', in Ellison, N. and Pierson, C. (eds) *Developments in British Social Policy*, London, Macmillan, pp. 173–87.

Mandleson, P. and Liddle, R. (1996) *The Blair Revolution: Can New Labour Deliver?* London, Faber & Faber.

Mannion, R. and Smith, P. (1998) 'How providers are chosen in the mixed economy of community care', in Bartlett, W., Roberts, J.A. and Le Grand, J. (eds) *A Revolution in Social Policy: Quasi-market Reforms in the 1990s*, Bristol, Policy Press, pp. 111–31.

Marsh, D. and Rhodes, R.A.W. (eds) (1992) *Implementing Thatcherite Policies: Audit of an Era*, Buckingham, Open University Press.

Marvin, S. and Guy, S. (1997) 'Smart metering technologies and privatised utilities', *Local Economy*, August, 119–32.

Maynard, A. (1988) 'Privatising the National Health Service', in C. Johnson (ed.) *Lloyds Bank Annual Review: Privatization and Ownership*, pp. 47–59.

Maynard, A. (1995) 'Reforming the NHS', in Bishop, M., Kay, J. and Mayer, C. (eds) *The Regulatory Challenge*, Oxford, Oxford University Press, pp. 67–83.

Mays, N. and Dixon, J. (1998) 'Purchaser plurality in UK healthcare: is a consensus emerging and is it the right one?', in Bartlett, W., Roberts, J.A. and Le Grand, J. (eds) *A Revolution in Social Policy: Quasi-market Reforms in the 1990s*, Bristol, Policy Press, pp. 175–99.

Meacher, M. (1985) *The Proposed Social Fund*, Birmingham, British Association of Social Workers.

Means, R. and Langan, J. (1996) 'Charging and quasi-markets in community care: implications for elderly people with dementia', in *Social Policy and Administration*, **30**(3), 244–62.

Miliband, D. (1990) *Markets, Politics and Education: Beyond the Education Reform Act*, London, IPPR.

Mitchell, J. (1990) 'Britain: privatisation as myth?', in Richardson, J.J. (ed.) *Privatisation and Deregulation in Canada and Britain*, Dartmouth, IRPP, pp. 15–36.

Mohan, D. (1986) 'Commercial medicine and the NHS in South East England: the shape of things to come?', in Eyles, J. (ed.) *Health Care and the City*, pp. 41–64, London: Occasional Paper 28, Department of Geography, Queen Mary College.

Moran, M. (1998) 'Explaining the rise of the market in health care', in Ranade, W. (ed.) *Markets and Health Care: A Comparative Analysis*, London, Longman, pp. 17–33.

Moran, M. and Prosser, T. (eds) (1994) *Privatization and Regulatory Change in Europe*, Buckingham, Open University Press.

Morgan, P. (ed.) (1995) *Privatisation and the welfare state: implications for consumers and the workforce*, Aldershot, Dartmouth.

MORI (1995) *Electricity Services: The Customer Perspective*, London, MORI.

National Audit Office (1990) *The Elderly: Information Requirements for Supporting the Implications Personal Pensions for the National Insurance Fund*, HCS5, London, HMSO.

National Children's Bureau (1996) 'Four Year Olds in Schools: What is Appropriate Provision?' *Childfacts*, London, National Children's Bureau.

National Consumer Council (1994) *Paying the Price: A Consumer View of Water, Gas, Electricity and Telephone Regulation*, London, NCC.

National Council for Voluntary Organisations (1989) *Summary of Government's Proposals for Community Care*, London.

National Housing Forum (1997) *Living Places: sustainable homes, sustainable communities*, London, National Housing Forum.

National Local Government Forum Against Poverty (1995) *Briefing Paper: Prepayment Water Devices*, London.

No Turning Back Group (1993) *Who Benefits? Re-inventing Social Security*, London, Conservative Political Centre.

North, N. (1998) 'Implementing strategy: the politics of healthcare commissioning', *Policy and Politics*, **26**(1), 5–14.

Nozick, R. (1974) *Anarchy, State and Utopia*, Oxford, Blackwell.

OFT (1996) *Health Insurance Report*, East Molesey, Office of Fair Trading.

Ofwat (1995) *Budget Payment Units*, letter from Director General, June 1995, London, OFWAT.

Oppenheim, C. and Lister, R. (1996) 'Ten years after the 1986 Social Security Act', in May, M., Brunsdon, E. and Craig, G. (eds) *Social Policy Review*, **8**, London, Social Policy Association.

Osborne, D. and Gaebler, T. (1992) *Reinventing Government: How the Entrepreneurial Spirit is Transforming the Public Sector*, Reading, Mass., Addison-Wesley.

Papadakis, E. and Taylor-Gooby, P. (1987) *The Private Provision of Public Welfare: State, Market and Community*, Brighton, Wheatsheaf.

Pearson, M. (1992) 'Health policy under Thatcher: pushing the market to the limits?', in Cloke, P. (ed.) *Policy and Change in Thatcher's Britain*, Oxford, Pergamon Press, pp. 215–46.

Pennance, F.G. and Gray, H. (1968) *Choice in Housing*, London, Institute of Economic Affairs.

Personal Social Services Research Unit (1997) *Eligibility Criteria for Social Services for Older People in England*, PSSRU, University of Manchester.

Piachaud, D. (1996) 'Means-testing and the Conservatives', *Benefits*, 15.

Pirie, M. and Butler, E. (1995) *The Fortune Account: the successor to social welfare*, London, Adam Smith Institute.

Plumridge, A. (1996) 'The privatisation of social housing', in Braddon, D. and Foster D. (eds) *Privatisation: Social Science Themes and Perspectives*, Aldershot, Dartmouth.

Powell, M. (1996) 'Granny's footsteps, fractures and the principles of the NHS', *Critical Social Policy*, **47**, 27–44.

Ranade, W. (1997) *A Future for the NHS? Health Care for the Millennium*, London, Longman.

Ranade, W. (ed.) (1998) *Markets and Health Care: A Comparative Analysis*, London, Longman.

Ranson, S. (1990) 'From 1944 to 1988: education, citizenship and democracy', in Flude, M. and Hammer, M. (eds) *The Education Reform Act, 1988: Its Origins and Implications*, Basingstoke, Falmer Press, pp. 1–20.

Rhodes, R.A.W. (1992) 'Changing intergovernmental relations', in Cloke, P. (ed.) *Policy and Change in Thatcher's Britain*, Oxford, Pergamon Press, pp. 55–76.

Ribbins, P. and Sherratt, B. (1997) *Radical Educational Policies and Conservative Secretaries of State*, London, Cassell.

Ritchie, J.H. (1994) *The report of the inquiry into the care and treatment of Christopher Clunis*, London, HMSO.

Roberts, J.A., Le Grand, J. and Bartlett, W. (1998) 'Lessons from experience of quasi-markets in the 1990s', in Bartlett, W., Roberts, J.A. and Le Grand, J. (1998) *A Revolution in Social Policy: Quasi-market Reforms in the 1990s*, Bristol, Policy Press, pp. 275–90.

Robinson, R. (1998) Efficiency and the NHS: A Case for Internal Markets, London, Institute for Economic Affairs.

Rowlingson, K. and Kempson, E. (1993) *Gas Debt and Disconnection*, London, Policy Studies Institute.

Rowlingson, K., Whyley, C., Newburn, T. and Berthoud, R. (1997) *Social Security Fraud: The Role of Penalties*, DSS Research Report 64, London, HMSO.

Ruane, S. (1997) 'Private-public boundaries and the transformation of the NHS', *Critical Social Policy*, **51**, 53–78.

Salter, B. (1995) 'The private sector and the NHS: redefining the welfare state', *Policy and Politics*, **23**(1), 17–30.

Seldon, A. (1981) *Wither the Welfare State*, London, IEA.

Sen, A. (1982) *Choice, Welfare and Measurement*, Oxford, Blackwell.

Sexton, S. (1987) *Our Schools – A Radical Policy*, London, IEA.

Sheffield Business School (1994) *Electricity, Self Disconnection Policy Initiatives and Informed Opinion: A Study*, Sheffield.

Shelter (1998) *Benefit Shortfalls: The Impact of Housing Benefit Cuts on Young Single People*, London, Shelter.

Shelter Cymru/Chartered Institute of Housing in Wales (1996) *Housing: The Key Issue*, Swansea, Shelter Cymru.

Silburn, R. (1992) 'The changing landscape of poverty', in Manning, N. and Page, R. (eds) *Social Policy Review*, **4**, London, Social Policy Association, pp. 134–53.

Sinfield, A. (1991) 'Why some are more secure than others', *Benefits*, September/October, 2–5.

Smee, C. (1995) 'Self-governing trusts and GP fundholders: the British experience', in Saltmann, R. and Von Otter, C. (eds) *Planned Markets and Public Competition*, Buckingham, Open University Press.

Smith, K.B. and Meier, K.J. (1995) *The Case Against School Choice: Politics, Markets and Fools*, Armonk, New York, M.E. Sharpe.

Smith, R., Walker, R. and Williams, P. (1996) 'Empowering the consumer: the case of social housing', in Morgan, P. (ed.) *Privatisation and the Welfare State: Implications for Consumers and the Workforce*, Aldershot, Dartmouth.

Smith, S.R. (1996) 'Transforming the public services: contracting for social and health services in the US', *Public Administration*, **74**, 113–27.

Smith, T. and Noble, M. (1995) *Education Divides: Poverty and Schooling in the 1990s*, London, CPAG.

Social Exclusion Unit (1998a) *Rough Sleeping Report*, Cm 4008, London, HMSO.

Social Exclusion Unit (1998b) *Truancy and School Exclusion Report*, London, HMSO.

Social Security Advisory Committee (1988) *Report*, London, HMSO.

Social Security Advisory Committee (1995) *Report*, Cm 2858, London, HMSO.

Stewart, G. (1998) 'Housing, poverty and social exclusion', in Shaw, I., Lambert, S. and Clapham, D. (eds) *Social Care and Housing*, London, Jessica Kingsley, pp. 47–62.

Stewart, J. and Clarke, M. (1987) 'The Public Service Orientation: issues and dilemmas', *Public Administration*, **69**(2) 161–77.

Sullivan, M. (1996) *Modern Social Policy*, London, Harvester Wheatsheaf.

Taylor-Gooby, P. (1993) 'The new educational settlement: National Curriculum and local management', in Taylor-Gooby, P. and Lawson, R. (eds) *Markets and Managers*, Buckingham, Open University Press, pp. 102–16.

Taylor-Gooby, P. (1998) 'No choice for poor pupils', *The Guardian*, 10 September.

Thompson, S. and Hoggett, P. (1996) 'Universalism, selectivism and particularism: towards postmodern social policy', *Critical Social Policy*, **46**, 21–43.

Timmins, N. (1996) *The Five Giants: A Biography of the Welfare State*, London, Fontana.

Titmuss, R.M. (1958) *Essays on the Welfare State*, London, Allen & Unwin.

Townsend, P., Davidson, N. and Whitehead, M. (1988) *Inequalities in Health*, Harmondsworth, Penguin Books.

Treasury (1995) *Public Expenditure*, Cmd. 2821, London, HMSO.

United Nations (1995) *Comparative Experiences with Privatisation: Policy Insights and Lessons Learned*, New York, United Nations.

Utility Week (1996) 'Prepayment and self-disconnection', 9 September.

Utting, W. (1997) *People Like Us: The Report of the Review of Safeguards for Children Living Away from Home*, London, Department of Health.

Veljanovski, C.G. (1987) *Selling the State: Privatisation in Britain*, London, Weidenfeld & Nicolson.

Vickers, J. and Wright, V. (eds) (1989) *The Politics of Privatisation in Western Europe*, London, Cass.

Vickers, J. and Yarrow, G. (1988) *Privatisation: An Economic Analysis*, Cambridge, Mass., MIT Press.

Waddhams-Price, C. (1997) 'Regulating for fairness: competition in the utilities can hurt the poor unless great care is taken', *New Economy*, **4**(2), 117–22.

Waine, B. (1995) 'A disaster foretold? The case of the personal pension', *Social Policy and Administration*, **29**(4), 317–34.

Waldegrave, W. (1987) *Some Reflections on Housing Policy*, Conservative Party News Service, 19 May.

Walker, R. (1997) 'New public management and housing associations', *Policy and Politics*, **26**(1), 71–88.

Walker, R. and Park, J. (1998) 'Unpicking poverty', in Oppenheim, C. (ed.) *An Inclusive Society: Strategies for Tackling Poverty*, London, IPPR, pp. 29–52.

Wall, A. (1996) 'Mine, yours or theirs? Accountability in the new NHS', *Policy and Politics*, **24**(1), 73–84.

Ward, S. (ed.) (1987) *Of Little Benefit*, London, Social Security Consortium.

Webb, A., Day, L. and Weller, D. (1976) *Voluntary Social Service Manpower Resources*, London, Personal Social Services Council.

Webster, C. (1988) *The Health Services since the War. Vol. 1, Problems of Health Care: The National Health Service before 1957*, London, HMSO.

Webster, C. (1998) *The National Health Service: A Political History*, Oxford, Oxford University Press.

West, E.G. (1996) 'Education without the state', in Seldon, A. (ed.) *Re-Privatising Welfare After the Lost Century*, London, Institute of Economic Affairs, pp. 11–19.

Whelan, R. (ed.) (1998) *Octavia Hill and the Social Housing Debate*, London, Institute of Economic Affairs.

Whitehead, M. (1994) 'Is it fair?: evaluating the equity implications of the NHS reforms', in Robinson, R. and Le Grand, J. (eds) *Evaluating the NHS Reforms*, Hermitage, King's Fund Institute.

Whiteside, N. (1998) 'Private agencies and public purposes: a quasi-market in the inter-war years', in Bartlett, W., Roberts, J.A. and Le Grand, J. (eds) *A Revolution in Social Policy: Quasi-market Reforms in the 1990s*, Bristol, Policy Press, pp. 201–16.

Whitty, G., Power, S. and Halpin, D. (1998) 'Self-managing schools in the market place: the experience of England, the USA and New Zealand', in Bartlett, W., Roberts, J.A. and Le Grand, J. (1998) *A Revolution in Social Policy: quasi-market reforms in the 1990s*, Bristol, Policy Press, 63–77.

Wilcox, S. (1996) *Housing Finance Review 1996/97*, York, Joseph Rowntree Foundation.

Wilcox, S. (1997a) 'Dwellings and households', in *Housing Finance Review 1997/98*, York, Joseph Rowntree Foundation, pp. 43–5.

Wilcox, S. (1997b) *Housing Finance Review 1997/98*, York, Joseph Rowntree Foundation.

Wilcox, S. and Ford, J. (1997) 'At your own risk', in Wilcox, S. (ed.) *Housing Finance Review 1997/98*, York, Joseph Rowntree Foundation, pp. 24–9.

Williams, P. (1992) 'Housing', in Cloke, P. (ed.) *Policy and Change in Thatcher's Britain*, Oxford, Pergamon Press, pp. 159–98.

Wistow, G. (1997) 'Funding long-term care', *Social Policy Review*, **9**.

Wistow, G. and Henwood, M. (1991) 'Caring for people: elegant model or flawed design?', in Manning, N. (ed.) *Social Policy Review 1990–91*, London, Longman.

Wright, D. (1997) *Are Local Authorities Avoiding Paying for Residential Care of Older People?*, London, Help the Aged.

Wright, V. (ed.) (1994) *Privatisation in Western Europe: Pressures, Problems and Paradoxes*, London, Printer Publishers.

Young, S. (1986) 'The nature of privatisation in Britain 1979–1985', *West European Politics*, **9**, 235–52.

NAME INDEX

This index contains the names of authors of academic and other reference texts who are cited in the text. The main index contains the names of those individuals who appear in the book as actors in their own right.

Ford 60, 61, 66
Forrest 7, 51, 52, 54, 56, 62, 64, 65
Foster 20
Fraser 9
Furbey 58

Gaebler 25
Garnham 79
Gewirtz 97, 100
Giddens 104
Gladstone 17
Glatter 93, 96, 97
Glennerster 14, 67, 88, 90, 95, 97, 139
Goldsmith 123
Goodwin 66
Graham 37, 43, 44
Grantovetter 131
Gray 55, 100
Green 15
Greer 78, 79
Guy 41, 42

Haines 72
Hall 151, 183, 186
Halpen 92
Ham 132
Hammer 86, 89, 91, 92
Harding 83
Hargreaves 86
Harriott 65
Harris 29, 31
Harrison 120
Hartley 18
Hayden 101
Heald 22, 23, 24
Hendry 6, 11
Henwood 106, 107, 113
Herbert 43
Hills 7, 8, 117, 67, 139, 149, 183, 184
Hirsch 98
Hirschman 23
Hoggett 23, 28, 30, 32
Houghton 44, 45
Hoyes 112
Huby 70, 71
Hunter 128, 131
Hutton 40, 151, 152
Hyams-Parish 101

Jack 83
Jacques 183
Jenkins 78
Jonathan 98
Joseph 12
Jowell 62
Judge 15

Kay 21
Kemp 54, 55, 56, 57, 60, 64
Kempson 43, 44, 61, 116
Kendall 104
Kirkpatrick 26
Knights 79

Labour Research 37, 95
Laing 105, 107
Land 77
Langan 111, 112
Lapsley 107
Le Grand 32, 110, 154
Lees 104
Letwin 22
Levenson 123
Lewis 109, 110, 111, 112, 113
Liddle 147
Linneman 6, 22, 25
Lister 71, 73
Llewellyn 107
Lloyd 148
Loughlin 25, 27
Lowe 67, 103
Lucio 26
Lund 53, 54, 56, 58, 63
Lunt 105, 107, 115, 116

Malpass 7, 59, 61, 63, 64, 66
Mandleson 147
Mannion 108, 110, 131
Marsh 21
Marvin 42
Matthews 15, 65
Maynard 119, 121, 126, 128, 132, 133
Meacher 70
Means 111, 112
Meier 100
Micklewright 69, 74, 75
Miliband 28, 91, 96, 98
Mitchell 28

GENERAL INDEX

Adam Smith Institute
  and case managers 112
  and G.P. fundholders 129
  and grant maintained schools 92
  and housing policy 55
  and open enrolment 99
  and social security reform 75
Anti-Social Behaviour Orders
  and Labour housing policy 143–4
  and social authoritarianism 144
Armstrong, H. 139, 140, 141
Audit Commission 93, 99, 112, 129

Baker, K. 92
Bevan, A. 129
  and health service principles 16, 118,
    119
  and *In Place of Fear* 190–1
  and resignation as health service
    minister 17
Beveridge 16, 129
  and Beveridge Report 189–90
  and Fabianism 29
  and Fowler Reviews 69
  and funeral expenses and 9, 10
  and Memorial Lecture by Frank Field
    148, 149
  and social security and 9
  and voluntarism and 13, 14
  New Labour abandonment of 146,
    149, 156
Blair, T. 4
  and importance of education policy 157
  and limits of willingness to fund
    welfare through taxation 147
  and New Deal for Regeneration
    145–6

and payment-by-results for teachers
    161
  and 'problem of welfare' 5
  and Rough Sleepers Initiative 144–5
  and sacking of Harriet Harman and
    Frank Field 148
  and social authoritarianism 152,
    185–6
  and *The Will To Win* 203–4
  and 'work for those who can' 149
  social security as part of problem not
    solution 146
Blunkett, D. 157
  and embrace of marketisation in
    education 161–3
  and New Labour education policy
    205–6
  and PFI 164
  as Secretary of State for Education
    157–9
  rejects poverty as source of
    underachievement 159
Bottomley, V. 116
  and health service reforms 194

Callaghan, J. 12
Communitarianism 152–3
Comprehensive Spending Review 140,
    145–6, 171, 174, 181
Conservative Party
  and 1987 General Election Manifesto
    192–3
Cox, Lady Caroline 12

Darling, A. 151
  and New Labour social security policy
    206–8

and Fowler Reviews 69–70, 73, 76
  and funeral expenses 81–3
  and privatisation of poverty 72
  and Social Fund 69–71
and housing benefit 63, 64, 72
and purchaser/provider relations 25
and reform of funeral payments 80–4
  and Castle Morpeth Council 83–4
and shifting burden of housing costs
    61
and young people and benefits 72, 81
early development of 9
fundamental to contract between
    individual and state 8
New Labour and 146–56
  and abandonment of Beveridge
      principles 146, 184
  and claimed erosion in public
      support for 148–9
  and obsession with fraud 154–5
  and pension reform 155–6, 184
  and privatisation of BAMS 146
  and redistribution of responsibility
      for 149, 151, 152, 156
  and stakeholding 153–4
  and triumph of 'neo-conservatism'
      in 151–2
  New Labour's preference for means-
      testing in 150–1, 156
occupational welfare and 10
Orme Review and 10
Personal pensions 76–8, 182
Peter Lilley and sectoral reform 73–5
shift of responsibility from public to
    private by 1997 84–5
trends between 1945 and 1979 10
Social Security Advisory Committee
  and *State Benefits and Private Provision*
    195–6
casts doubt on claims for privatisation
    77
objects to changes in funeral expense
    payments 81
Social Services
  and charging policy 105
    and community care 106–16
      and Direct Payment scheme 116
      and distortion of demand for 116,
        172

and equity impact of 115, 166,
    171
and health/social services
    boundary 106–7
and pressures on local
    government to recover costs
    through 114–15
and variable pattern of charging
    in 116, 166, 171, 172
and contract culture 108–10
and private residential care 105–6,
    127, 168, 169
and Conservative inheritance in 1979
    103–4
and Direct Payment scheme 116–17,
    172
and Griffiths Report 106, 107, 109
and New Labour 162–72
and private insurance for costs in later
    life 116–17
and providing services 111–14
  and attitudes of voluntary and for-
      profit providers 113–14
  and co-option of senior managers
      114
and rationing and the individual
    arbitrary outcomes of 114, 116
    case for 114
    equity deficits in relation to 115
    impact on poorest consumers 115,
      116
early origins of 13
enduring mixed economy within 14,
    103, 117, 165
non-universal character of 103, 117
rejected by New Labour 172
Seebohm Report and 14
voluntary provision of 13, 14
Stakeholding 153–4
  and stakeholder pensions 155–6

Thatcher, M.
  absence of interest in homelessness 64
  and dislike of consensus 121
  and dislike of local authorities 108
  and economic freedom and social
      control 104
  and encouragement of private
      medicine 124